PENGUIN HANDBOOKS

MIND OVER LABOR

Carl Jones is the author of *Sharing Birth: A Father's Guide to Giving Support During Labor* and *After the Baby Is Born*. A certified childbirth educator, he lives in New Hampshire with his wife, Jan, and their three sons, Carl, Paul, and Jonathan.

D1053934

⮴ CARL JONES

Mind Over Labor

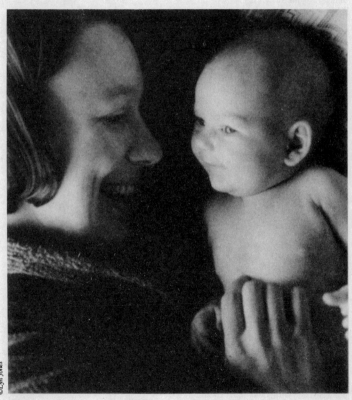

©Lyn Jones

PENGUIN BOOKS

PENGUIN BOOKS
Viking Penguin Inc., 40 West 23rd Street,
New York, New York 10010, U.S.A.
Penguin Books Ltd, 27 Wrights Lane, London W8 5TZ
(Publishing & Editorial) and Harmondsworth,
Middlesex, England (Distribution & Warehouse)
Penguin Books Australia Ltd, Ringwood,
Victoria, Australia
Penguin Books Canada Limited, 2801 John Street,
Markham, Ontario, Canada L3R 1B4
Penguin Books (N.Z.) Ltd, 182–190 Wairau Road,
Auckland 10, New Zealand

First published in the United States of America by
Viking Penguin Inc. 1987
Published in Penguin Books 1988

Grateful acknowledgment is made for permission to reprint an excerpt
from "Little Gidding" in *Four Quartets* by T. S. Eliot. Copyright 1936
by Harcourt Brace Jovanovich, Inc.; copyright © 1963, 1964 by T. S. Eliot.
Reprinted by permission of Harcourt Brace Jovanovich, Inc.,
and Faber and Faber Ltd.

LIBRARY OF CONGRESS CATALOGING IN PUBLICATION DATA
Jones, Carl.
  Mind over labor.
  Bibliography: p.
  Includes index.
  1. Natural childbirth.   2. Imagery (Psychology)
3. Mind and body.   I. Title.
[RG661.J579   1988]   618.4'5   87-7126
ISBN 0 14 046.762 9

Printed in the United States of America by
R. R. Donnelley & Sons Company, Harrisonburg, Virginia
Set in Goudy Old Style
Designed by Vicky Hartman

To Carl and Paul

Foreword by
Emmett E. Miller, M.D.

Few books in the field of health care have the potential to be epoch-making. *Mind Over Labor* is one of them. This highly effective guide is a milestone in a newly emerging approach to childbirth.

Today the old images and models of childbearing are giving place to a new model. There is a growing groundswell of awareness that birth is a point of maximum power for women. We are moving away from rigid structures and styles of breathing. We are moving toward a more holistic approach to labor.

Mind Over Labor leads the way. In the vanguard of holistic health care, this book introduces a breakthrough method of childbirth preparation based on using the mind's power to reduce the fear and pain of labor.

More and more health professionals in all fields are turning to relaxation and mental imagery—a means of turning thoughts into inner pictures. In my own practice as a family physician and specialist in psychophysiological medicine, I have found imagery extremely effective in treating a wide spectrum of health problems, including lowering high blood pressure, gaining control over tension and migraine headaches, and helping women reduce the pain of labor as well as lessen their chances of childbirth-related complications.

Mind Over Labor shows how the dynamic technique of mental

imagery can play a key role in a unique childbirth preparation method any woman and her partner can follow with minimum effort. The eight-step method this book outlines will prove a far more effective coping tool than breathing patterns for most child-bearing couples.

This inspiring, beautifully written volume offers childbearing couples a fresh perspective on labor. *Mind Over Labor* shows in simple, moving terms how labor is an event of the mind as well as of the body. It shows couples how, by acknowledging this fact, they can make birth the wonderful, enriching experience it can be for mother, father, and child. It inspires self-confidence, self-esteem, self-acceptance. *Mind Over Labor* encourages a woman to believe in her own power, which is, after all, what brings a child into the world.

In my own practice, I am continually reminded how a negative image of birth can create a longer, more difficult labor and some-times lead to complications. So many labors are made overpainful by self-doubt and fear. Potentially beautiful birthing experiences are ruined by frightening images. *Mind Over Labor* shows couples how to release harmful, inappropriate, and potentially destruc-tive beliefs that could otherwise inhibit normal labor. At the same time, it encourages couples to be themselves rather than conform to an outside model.

In an era when childbearing couples and health professionals have allowed themselves to become overdependent on technol-ogy, this book is more than welcome. It emphasizes birth as a normal, natural event—a sexual process rather than a medical crisis. In many ways it represents a rediscovery of ideas that sensitive, observant birth attendants in cultures throughout the world have known for centuries—for example, that the emotions and environment influence the childbearing process. But never before have these ideas been presented in such a usable fashion and stated so clearly, so simply, and so insightfully.

In presenting the mental-imagery techniques, Carl Jones draws on the experience of scientists as well as laypersons. He also adds his own special insight.

It is refreshing to find a book like this written by a male childbirth educator. When my wife and I first attended Lamaze classes, preparing for the birth of our son, I had the feeling of being swallowed up in a world of women. Traditionally, women have written about the emotional and men about the technical aspects of birth. Carl Jones does both. A pioneer childbirth professional, he has proved that a man can understand not only the technical side of obstetrics but the experience of childbirth as well. This in itself is a breakthrough.

Mind Over Labor is not just a book to be read but something to be experienced. I wholeheartedly recommend it to everyone planning to have a baby.

Emmett E. Miller, M.D.,
author of *Self-Imagery: Creating Your Own Good Health* and the
Software for the Mind series
of cassette tape recordings

Foreword by
Marian Tompson

Little did I realize, when the manuscript of *Mind Over Labor* arrived in the mail, that it would play an important role during the labor that preceded the birth of my tenth grandchild, Matthew Colin Fagerholm. My daughter Allison had phoned earlier in the day to announce that her labor had started. As I tossed a few things into a bag, I took the manuscript along, too.

Allison and Michael had planned very carefully for the event, reading books, choosing the right physician, and faithfully attending childbirth classes. Allison was also very careful to eat nutritiously. Though this was her first pregnancy, she had helped out during the labors of her sisters. Birth was no mystery to her.

But Allison's labor turned out to be different from those of her four sisters. The baby's position presented a problem, and after twenty-four hours of active labor, the contractions started slowing down. Finally we decided to transfer to the hospital. Yet contractions still did not pick up. After Allison and Michael had tried a number of techniques to deal with the situation, we decided to try an imagery exercise described in *Mind Over Labor*. We chose *The Opening Flower*, an imagery especially effective when dilatation slows down or stops. Using a light, caressing massage, we kept repeating the scenario of walking in a garden and concentrating on the unfolding of a particular rose, while Allison immersed herself in the images.

And it worked! Matthew was born healthy. Later, Allison realized that never once during her long, difficult labor did she feel the need for any kind of painkiller. Using mental imagery at that critical point, along with the continuous support of her husband and the reassuring presence of her physician, gave her what she needed to carry on so superbly.

. There are many books available on childbirth today, but none that I know of focuses so well on the influence of our thoughts and emotions on childbirth as does *Mind Over Labor*. Carl Jones provides a fresh perception of the needs of the pregnant woman. He sheds light on those factors, sometimes very subtle, that can enhance or impede her birth experience.

Yet it is an easy book to read. This clear, simple, practical eight-step guide shows how mental imagery can be used to advantage, starting in pregnancy, and how this preparation will prove valuable even when unexpected complications arise. The tools Carl Jones offers are especially helpful for first-time mothers, but they are also helpful for the woman who has had a disappointing experience with a previous birth.

There is something else special about *Mind Over Labor*. This is Carl Jones's own background as both a childbirth educator and the father of three boys, one born in the hospital, two at home. While he rarely calls attention to his own perspective, his personal experience comes through in his practical, down-to-earth presentation of eight steps for a rewarding birth. Carl Jones understands that special attunement a woman has with her unborn baby. He knows the kind of support a laboring woman needs from her mate. He understands the feelings and needs of the father as well as those of the mother during the childbearing experience.

One of the most powerful moments of my grandchild Matthew's birth actually occurred when he was placed in his father's arms. During Allison's pregnancy, Michael talked to Matthew daily. During the birth Matthew emerged rather precipitously after a second stage that had gone on for hours. His startled crying reflected his shock and bewilderment. When he was wrapped in a blanket, handed to his father, and heard Michael's voice, the character of his crying changed immediately to one of relief after a scare. And Allison and I, watching with tears in our eyes, knew that Matthew was telling his father how hard he had tried to be born and how happy he was finally to be held by his dad. Matthew knew who his father was, and in that profound moment Michael also knew how important he was to his son.

So thank you, Carl Jones, for adding to our insights on how we may best determine and meet our needs during childbirth. For it is only when we truly understand the intricacies of the childbearing process that we will be able to create a system of maternity care that will assure all couples the kind of support they need to get their families off to the best possible start.

> Marian Tompson,
> co-author of *The Womanly Art of Breastfeeding*,
> co-founder of La Leche League International

Contents

Mind Over Labor

CHAPTER ONE

Mind Over Labor

What will my labor be like? No doubt you wonder. Will I be able to handle it? Will I give birth normally? Most expectant mothers ask themselves such questions.

Labor can be a nightmare of agony and confusion. Or it can be a fulfilling experience—potentially one of the most fulfilling life has to offer.

The choice is yours.

This book will show you how to create the kind of birth you want.

The method outlined in the chapters ahead combines commonsense planning, relaxation, and mental imagery—a tool to bring about a desired result by translating positive thoughts into dynamic mental images. This method is based on two ideas which, taken together, spell one of the most significant breakthroughs in childbirth:

1. The mind influences childbirth in a remarkable way, and
2. Using mental imagery can alter the course of labor.

Many people have the idea, often mistaken, that some women's bodies are better adapted to giving birth than others. Or they imagine that only brave women can enjoy a natural birth.

But in the absence of unusual complications every woman can have a safe, fulfilling natural birth.

As often as not the cause of an overly long or unusually painful labor is to be found not in the mother's body but in the mind, the emotions. When it comes to childbirth complications, frequently it's the mind, not the body, that impairs normal labor.

Today as never before, childbirth professionals realize that labor works best *when mind and body cooperate.* No method of childbirth preparation can be completely successful unless this fact is taken into account.

Birth is the most significant biological, emotional, and social event you and your baby will share. Whether or not you and your baby have a happy birth depends largely on your preparation of the mind as well as the body. The steps you take now, during pregnancy, to prepare your mind and body influence the degree of pain, the length of labor, your birth experience, and even the way you feel after the baby is born.

Mind Over Labor consists of eight simple steps that anyone can follow. Discussed thoroughly in the chapters ahead, these are:

1. Understanding the "inner event of labor," that is the psychological and emotional dimensions of the labor process
2. Developing a positive image of birth
3. Relaxing body and mind
4. Using mental imagery during pregnancy
5. Creating the optimal birthing environment
6. Inviting attendants to your birth with whom you feel comfortable
7. Using mental imagery in labor
8. Enjoying the first hour after birth together

These steps will *reduce the pain and fear of labor* and in many cases actually shorten labor as well. *Mind Over Labor* does not promise painless childbirth. However, this method will open the door for you to experience a safe, rewarding birth—the birth you truly desire.

You can expect a host of benefits from using the eight-step method outlined on the pages ahead. The method will enable you to:

- Be more relaxed
- Enjoy a more fulfilling pregnancy
- Be more aware of your baby's and your needs
- Be attuned to your unborn child
- Create or strengthen a positive image of birth
- Choose the optimal caregiver
- Relate to your caregiver with confidence
- Choose the optimal birthing place
- Reduce the pain and fear of labor
- Cope with labor smoothly
- Maximize your partner's ability to give you effective labor support
- Lessen the chance of tearing during birth
- Deal effectively with specific variations in labor such as prolonged or overdue labor
- Lessen the chance of a cesarean and other complications
- Reduce the chance of postpartum blues
- Assist the process of breastfeeding

The Mind/Body Process of Childbirth

An explosion of new discoveries has revealed startling facts about how the mind influences the body. Numerous studies have shown that the state of our health reflects our mental attitudes. Holistic health care (any of several branches of medicine emphasizing the whole person) has given medical researchers new perspectives on the many ways emotions, thoughts, and beliefs influence physical processes.

Biofeedback research has proved that one can control bodily processes once thought to be entirely involuntary, such as heartbeat, blood pressure, and even brain waves, with the use of mental imagery—that is, by forming relaxing images in the mind. A biofeedback machine monitors physiological processes through electrodes attached to the skin and makes them perceptible. With practice the person who is being monitored learns to exercise a surprising degree of control over these physiological processes.

Barbara Brown, a leader in the biofeedback field, states that medical researchers are "learning that relationships between mind and body are more powerful than they once thought." Though mental imagery has been used for healing throughout the world since ancient times, she claims that "research into biofeedback is the first medically testable indication that the mind can relieve illnesses as well as create them."[1]

Dr. Herbert Benson wrote in *The Relaxation Response* that patients with elevated blood pressure can learn to lower it by "thinking relaxing thoughts." At Beth Israel Hospital in Boston, he teaches patients a simple form of meditation that can bring about mental calmness to decrease hypertension.

Dr. Benson points out that those who practice yoga and zen can alter their metabolism and that those who meditate can "produce changes in the electrical activity of the brain."[2] Some have suggested that mental imagery affects the body's energy fields. Yogis and meditators have recognized the mind's ability to control involuntary bodily processes for thousands of years. But for Western medicine, the nature of the mind-body relationship is a recent discovery.

Labor and the Mind

Our knowledge of human labor and birth is far from complete. No one can determine exactly when a baby will be born—the estimated due date is accurate only 5 percent of the time. No one knows what causes labor to begin when it does. No one knows what keeps the uterus contracting at regular intervals once labor has begun. And no one can predict what a particular woman's labor will be like any more than one can guess the pattern of a snowflake before it falls.

But of one thing we are certain: *Labor is an event of the mind as well as the body.*

Of all our physical functions, only lovemaking is as much influenced by thoughts and emotion as labor. The way the mother thinks and feels affects the way she gives birth.

When it is time for the baby to be born the uterus will, of course, contract regardless of how a woman feels about labor. Her baby will be born whether she thinks positive thoughts or despises every minute of childbearing. But the way she thinks, feels, and believes will influence the discomfort and length of her labor—and the safety of birth for her and her baby.

Midwives have known for centuries that mind and body interact during childbearing. But only recently have studies *proved* the dramatic effects of mind over labor.

For example, studies have shown that laboring women who have their partners with them tend to have shorter, less painful labors. This is presumably because the partner's presence makes the mother feel more comfortable and secure. She is therefore better able to cope with labor.[3]

Similarly, women who have taken childbirth preparation classes appear to have shorter and less painful labors. Medication is used less often. The new mothers react more positively immediately after birth. One study shows that the average duration of labor was five hours shorter among women who attended classes than among others of the same socioeconomic class who had not taken classes.[4] Women who have been to childbirth preparation classes are better informed. They know what to expect in labor. As a result they are less afraid and more confident about giving birth.

Eye-opening studies show that altering one's beliefs about childbirth can actually shorten labor by as much as 25 to 50 percent.[5]

One of these studies compared two groups of women matched for age, number of previous births, use of medication, and so on. The first group prepared for birth using a method devised by Grantly Dick-Read, a British obstetrician who taught in the 1930s that labor was not meant to be painful, stressed the importance of relaxation and a positive attitude, and wrote about the joy and elation of the entire reproductive process, including birth. The other group of women were not familiar with Read's ideas. Significantly, the total duration of contractions among the Read-prepared women was 25 percent shorter than that of the other women.[6]

In another revealing study a group received the suggestion, under hypnosis, that labor would be easy. They were not told it would be short. However, the duration of labor among those who had received the suggestion was nearly 50 percent shorter than that of the control group. Apparently the belief that labor would not be difficult relieved much fear and possible emotional disturbance, enabling the women to relax—leading, in turn, to more efficient labor.[7]

The time of day a woman gives birth is also partly affected by the mind. Analyzing 601,222 normal labors, one study showed that the peak incidence of birth occurs between 3 and 4 A.M.[8] Researchers believe this is so because a woman feels most relaxed and undisturbed during the peaceful early morning hours. The peak incidence of the onset of labor also occurs at night.

Labor frequently slows down and sometimes even stops altogether upon admission to the hospital. Presumably the cause is anxiety: Upon moving to unfamiliar surroundings, the anxious mother stops her labor unconsciously. As Elizabeth Noble points out in *Childbirth With Insight,* "The uterus works involuntarily, but it is very sensitive to discord in the mother's body and mind. Labors can slow down and even stop in reaction to such things as a change in the external environment during admission to hospital or negative attitudes in outsiders, family, friends, or the mother herself."[9]

"It is not really surprising that anxiety can slow labor," writes Valmai Elkins in The Birth Report. "It has been a well-known fact for years in animal husbandry."[10]

Many childbirth professionals believe that there is also a greater proportion of complications among anxious women.[11] Niles Newton, professor in the department of psychiatry at Northwestern University and author of Maternal Emotions, found that disturbances in the environment had significant effects on laboring mice. A number of mice near delivery were moved every hour or two from a glass bowl with cat odor to a familiar sheltered cage, so that an equal number of mice were always in both the bowl or the cage. A far greater number of mice delivered in the sheltered cage.

In a similar study a group of laboring mice were disturbed by being held gently in the hand for one minute. The disturbance contributed to a 65–72 percent delay in labor.[12]

Dr. Newton also showed that the health of the offspring was affected by the mother's labor environment. She compared a group of laboring mice who were periodically moved from one glass bowl to another with another group allowed to be in a sheltered environment. Significantly, 54 percent more pups died in the glass bowl than in the sheltered environment.

We can assume that human mothers are far more sensitive to emotional disturbances and to their birthing environment than laboring mice.

Ways the Mind Influences Labor

We don't know—and probably will never know—all the ways the mind affects labor, or precisely how the mother's thoughts and emotions so powerfully influence childbearing. But we do know that thoughts and emotions influence the experience of birth as surely as does the mother's health.

Factors that affect labor include: fear; the mother's ability to trust her body and surrender to the labor process; her attitude about birth; her emotions regarding this particular birth; her feelings about parenthood; her feelings about sexuality; her birthing environment; and her caregiver and others in the environment.

These subjects are more fully discussed in the chapters ahead. For now let's take a brief glance at two of the most dramatic factors that influence labor: fear and the effect of hormones.

Fear

Fear can increase both the pain and the length of labor. During labor fear overstimulates the sympathetic (involuntary) nervous system that controls blood vessel contraction, heartbeat, sweating, and so on. This induces the muscles of the uterus to tighten around the cervix, causing the uterus to work more forcefully and longer to open the tight cervix. The increased tension produced within the uterine walls also results in increased discomfort.

The mother's fear can also affect the baby. "Fear decreases the amount of blood reaching the baby," writes Dr. Lewis Mehl, an expert on the psychophysiological dimensions of childbearing. "This can cause the baby to be very susceptible to fetal distress during labor due to the chronic problem with lack of oxygen. Fear can prevent or disrupt an effective uterine contraction pattern. This physiological response to fear makes sense in the animal kingdom. An animal uses this reflex to stop labor in the presence of danger. . . . For people, much of their fear is generated from images or thoughts rather than external events. The consequences can be just as physiological."[13]

The Effect of Hormones

An efficient labor depends on the right hormonal balance. The right hormonal balance is, in turn, influenced by emotions.

Oxytocin is one of the hormones responsible for regulating uterine contractions. It is released by the posterior pituitary gland during labor, nursing, and sexual arousal—three processes in a woman's life that require relaxation, comfort, and positive emotional feelings. "The release of oxytocin," Niles Newton observes, "is easily conditioned and inhibited by outside stimuli."[14]

This labor-regulating hormone also triggers "let-down," the milk-ejection reflex, during nursing. All health professionals are aware that oxytocin is released when the mother is relaxed and emotionally at ease, and that its release, and consequently the let-down reflex, can be impaired if the nursing mother feels inhibited or anxious. "Stresses such as embarrassment, irritation, or anxiety actually prevent the pituitary from secreting oxytocin," explains Karen Pryor in *Nursing Your Baby*.[15]

Certain hormones released under conditions of psychological stress can impair labor for both the mother and the baby. For example, stress-induced higher plasma cortisol levels have been linked to a longer first stage of labor. Higher levels of plasma epinephrine can cause a longer second stage. The stress-induced release of catecholamines and increased levels of adrenocorticoid steroids (as well as other hormones in the mother's circulation) can decrease uterine blood flow and the amount of oxygen the baby receives.[16]

We are still learning about how the mind influences labor. Meanwhile, hundreds of childbirth professionals throughout the country have discovered that acquiring knowledge of anatomy and learning how to breathe in a particular way are less important than developing confidence in the body and faith in the life-creating miracle. Today the emphasis in childbirth education is shifting from learning precise and rigid techniques to tapping inner resources that help the mother surrender to the labor process.

Mind Over Labor's eight-step method—based on the mind's influence on labor and the use of the power of mental imagery—will show you how to avoid anxiety-induced complications and to create the birth you truly desire.

The Power of Mental Imagery

Tapping the power of mental imagery—a method of using the mind to influence behavior and attain specific goals by translating positive thoughts into dynamic mental images—is an integral part of the eight-step method of this book. Enthusiasm for this subject is spreading like wildfire throughout the country. Mental imagery has kindled the excitement of professionals in a wide variety of fields and is used successfully in medicine, sports, business, clinical psychology, and education.

Carl and Stephanie Simonton, pioneers in the field of cancer therapy, have discovered that beliefs, attitudes, and feelings affect our overall health. Combining mental imagery with traditional medicine, they have had remarkable results in the treatment of cancer. Carl, a radiation oncologist who specializes in cancer treatment, and Stephanie, a psychotherapist, run the Cancer Counseling and Research Center in Dallas, Texas. Many of their patients are diagnosed "medically incurable" by other physicians, yet under the Simontons' care cancer patients have a recovery rate twice that of the national average. Many experience complete remissions. [17]

In the field of sports W. Timothy Gallwey's bestselling books *The Inner Game of Tennis* and *The Inner Game of Golf* focus not on physical techniques but on the player's mental image and inner development. Gallwey instructs tennis players to imagine hitting the ball where they want it to go, then to just let the body do it, let it happen.

In the business world mental imagery has opened the door to new methods of professional training and development. David Meier, director of the Center for Accelerated Learning, a training, consulting, and research firm in Lake Geneva, Wisconsin, states: "Imagery is the mother tongue of the deeper mind and a powerful internal force influencing the mind/body system." Among the uses of mental imagery in business, Meier lists learning, tapping inner wisdom and knowledge, problem solving, personal unfolding, and success patterning. "Professional development," he writes, "can never again denote simply the acquisition of external skills and techniques, but must include developing the full range of internal and spiritual skills as well."[18]

Childbirth education is just catching up. Hundreds of childbirth professionals throughout the country have recently discovered the power of mental imagery.

Mental Imagery and Childbirth

Deirdre, a university professor pregnant with her first child, was terrified of labor. She doubted that she could birth naturally. "I want to do it," she told her physician. "But it's just not possible for me."

Her physician, Dr. Emmett Miller, a pioneer in the field of psychophysiological medicine, suggested that Deirdre take five steps: (1) Relaxation practice. (2) Envisioning the child within so it "stopped being just a big belly and started to be a real child for her," then imagining herself with her baby after birth. (3) Letting go of frightening images (such as "babies getting stuck in the middle," "women bleeding to death," and so on) which Deirdre had picked up when very young. Dr. Miller asked her to look at these images objectively, recognizing that they were a product of the hysteria of people in her environment and they needn't concern her. (4) Envisioning the labor process. (5) Using supportive, positive suggestions such as "I'm confident in my ability to birth naturally," "The strength of my uterine contractions is a sign of my feminine strength," and "I love my child and I am capable of doing all that is necessary to bring about a healthy birth."

After having taken these steps, Deirdre's fears dissolved. Her unmedicated labor was very smooth. The birth was rewarding, "near ecstatic," with Deirdre smiling victorious when she cradled the child in her arms. After the baby was born, she said it felt like "pushing your team across the goal in the final few seconds of the Super Bowl—hard work but not painful!"

Aristotle's statement that "a vivid imagination compels the whole body to obey it" is probably nowhere more true than in childbearing. In fact, mental imagery is probably more suited to childbirth preparation than to any other endeavor.

"Mental imagery can actually bring about physiological changes and alter the course of labor," states Suzanna May Hilbers, Registered Physical Therapist and ASPO/Lamaze certified childbirth educator. (ASPO is the American Society of Psychoprophylaxis in Obstetrics.) After having taught the subject to hundreds of childbirth professionals and prospective parents, she considers mental imagery the most powerful method a couple can use to prepare for a fulfilling birth experience.

According to Dr. Emmett Miller, who has worked with mental imagery in childbirth preparation for the last fifteen years and is one of the nation's leading experts on the subject, using mental imagery in childbirth preparation can lead to "deep relaxation, flowing with rather than resisting the experience; a higher level of functioning; a less physically traumatic birth and more pain-free delivery; and less need for instrumentation and the use of anesthetic agents."

Hundreds of childbirth professionals working independently of one another have made similar discoveries.

"We use mental imagery to facilitate the progress of labor," states Loretta Ivory, a nurse midwife from Denver on the faculty of several universities. "And we've discovered that it does so quite dramatically!"

Janet Kingsepp, midwife and childbirth educator in eastern Texas who has taught mental imagery to over 250 couples, compares the method to the imaginary exercises Russian athletes do to program themselves for peak performance. In her practice she has found that mental imagery "definitely shortens labor." The results, she says, "depend on how much the client wants to put into it, how motivated she is. Most start out motivated by fear of labor. But as they use mental imagery, they later discover they can create the birth they want."

Detroit childbirth educator Rose Heman, registered nurse and co-founder of New Life Holistic Education Association, teaches physicians, midwives, nurses, and childbirth educators how to use mental imagery. Like Suzanna Hilbers, she believes that mental imagery is the most effective form of childbirth preparation, reducing the chance of complications and the need for medical intervention.

According to Barbara Pepper of the Midwifery Training Institute in Albuquerque, New Mexico, "Using mental imagery gives women a greater ability to enjoy pregnancy, the birth process, and the early postpartum." Most important, the method helps the mother "experience a psychological and physical openness as well as a sense of her own power."

How Does Mental Imagery Influence Labor?

Why is mental imagery so effective in pregnancy and labor? How does it work?

In a nutshell, mental imagery creates a smoother labor by promoting deep relaxation, helping you surrender to the process, and facilitating the release of labor-regulating hormones.

Following are some of the reasons this means of translating thoughts into dynamic images is so effective during the childbearing season:

- Mental imagery works with and influences the right hemisphere of the brain. This hemisphere is associated with intuition, emotion, lovemaking, and labor, and is often referred to as the *heart brain*. (The left hemisphere, on the other hand, is associated with analysis and intellectual pursuits.) During pregnancy and particularly during labor, the right hemisphere is more active than usual, while the left is less so. According to Dr. Miller, mental imagery translates cognitive information into terms that can activate the right hemisphere and actually help bring about the goal imagined.
- You are in close touch with your instinctive self and inner

resources during the transformative months of pregnancy. Mental imagery helps you tap these resources and attune to your instincts. By so doing, mental imagery encourages mind and body to cooperate during the childbearing process.

- During labor the mother enters a unique state of mind (discussed in chapter two) which is especially receptive to suggestion and imagery.

- Using mental imagery regularly during pregnancy often inspires practical changes in the mother's birth plans. As she focuses her mind on a desired goal, she may begin to think of concrete ways to bring about that goal (such as a different birthing place or caregiver).

- Using mental imagery may help clear away possible emotional hindrances that could inhibit normal labor.

Mental imagery will work most effectively when you are familiar with the physical and psychological dimensions of labor, understand the essentials of a positive image of birth, and learn to relax. Accordingly, we will turn to these subjects before going further into imagery.

Today most expectant parents want an emotionally rewarding birth in addition to a healthy mother and baby. You can have both. A safe birth and a fulfilling birth experience go hand in hand.

In the chapters that follow you will discover how to harness your physical, emotional, and spiritual resources to achieve the optimum birth experience.

The eight-step method requires minimal time and energy. However, it does require the open-mindedness to explore your feelings and look at new ideas, to reevaluate your image of birth. Other than that, all you need is the willingness to read the following chapters, try the exercises, and discover the most powerful tool you have in shaping a more fulfilling pregnancy and a safe, happy birth.

CHAPTER TWO

Understanding the Inner Event of Labor:
THE FIRST STEP

Insight is more important than knowledge when it comes to preparing for childbirth. This chapter will give you a fresh perspective on labor. By understanding the psychological, emotional, and sexual dimensions of labor (the *inner event of labor*) you will better prepare for birth.

The *inner event of labor* is largely the foundation for the eight steps in this book. A clear picture of this aspect of labor explains why steps such as creating the optimal birthing environment, choosing the right caregiver, and using mental imagery in labor will influence your birth.

We will explore the *inner event of labor* in detail after first discussing the physical process.

The Laboring Body

By the time labor begins the real work of childbearing—the creation of a new human being within your womb—has already taken place. Your body has accomplished a biological miracle. Your womb has provided the perfect conditions for your baby to grow from something smaller than the dot at the end of this sentence into the being you will soon cradle in your arms. Your body has created the placenta through which your unborn child receives everything he needs to develop. Your breasts are creating the only fully nutritious and safest food for your infant.

By comparison labor seems small business.

More ancient than medicine, birth is as old as organic life. Your body knows how to give birth just as your body knows how to provide for the needs of your growing baby within. For the most part, with the method in this book you will *create the conditions* for your body to labor optimally.

During labor the uterus rhythmically tightens and relaxes. The rhythmical tightenings called *contractions* occur intermittently until the baby and placenta (afterbirth) are born.

Labor contractions are often compared to ocean waves. Each surges, reaches a crest, and ebbs away. At the beginning of labor the waves are usually gentle, like little ripples. As labor unfolds they grow in intensity. Finally, toward labor's climax, they may seem furiously powerful like the waves of a stormy sea.

Labor has three stages. Though distinct, the stages of labor blend into one another.

First stage is the opening of the gateway. Contractions thin (efface) and open (dilate) the cervix little by little until it is wide enough for the baby to be born. Cervical dilation (sometimes spelled dilatation) is measured in centimeters. The cervix is fully dilated at about ten centimeters (four inches).

If you think of the uterus as an inverted pear with the stem protruding into the vagina, the cervix corresponds to the stem end. This is the uterine gateway, which admits the sperm at conception and will open for the baby to leave the womb during labor.

Before pregnancy the cervix is as hard as the tip of the nose, but hormones released as the baby grows soften it. During labor it is as soft as the earlobe and quite stretchable.

As dilation continues the contractions also push the baby downward so that the cervix begins to stretch over his head like the neck of a tight sweater.

First stage is more or less arbitrarily divided into three phases: *early* (0–4 cm.), *active* (4–7 cm.), and *transition* (7–10 cm.).

Contractions occur at increasingly shorter intervals as labor progresses. The frequency of contractions is measured from the beginning of one contraction to the beginning of the next. This means that if a sixty-second-long contraction occurs at 2:00 and another begins at 2:05, they are said to be occurring at five-minute intervals though the actual time between them is only four minutes.

During *early* labor (the cervix dilating to 4 cm.) contractions are generally mild, last from 30 to 45 seconds each, and occur about every 20 to 5 minutes. Contractions become more frequent as early labor blends into the active phase.

During *active* labor (cervix dilating to 7–8 cm.) contractions may last anywhere from 45 to 75 seconds each and occur every 7 to 2 minutes (the average being 5-to-3-minute intervals).

During the *transition* phase (cervix dilating fully to 10 cm.) contractions last 60 to 120 seconds and occur every 3 to 2 minutes. For many mothers this phase is the most difficult and they feel particularly vulnerable. Others don't notice a distinct transition phase.

Transition is really just a word to describe late active labor. Some childbirth educators dislike the word, believing there is really no separate transition phase. However, for many women transition is a qualitatively different part of labor with definite characteristics such as increased discomfort, irritability, tearfulness, and so forth.

First stage may last from two or three hours to thirty-six hours or longer. The average length is about twelve hours. Labor is usually, but not always, shorter for second-time mothers.

Bear in mind that there is a wide range of variation in normal labor. Your contractions may be totally different from those described above, yet be completely normal.

Second stage is the birth of the baby. It begins when the cervix is fully dilated. The mother usually feels an urge to bear down with contractions and push her baby out. Sometimes the urge to bear down comes shortly before full dilation and the mother will be asked not to bear down to avoid damage to the cervix.

At this point, while the work is far from over, the contractions usually feel different. They are usually less uncomfortable than those of first stage. For many, second stage is a positive, enjoyable part of labor. "I have never felt anything so marvelous," one mother said. "It cannot be compared to ordinary pleasure."[1] For others, however, it can be long and difficult. Women's experiences of second-stage labor range from "pushing was exquisite pleasure," "a relief," "exhilarating!" to "miserable!" "the hardest part of my labor."

In any case, most would agree that this is the most exciting and dramatic part of the childbearing miracle. The mother greets her child. The baby's head moves down during, and slips back between, contractions, making a little progress each time. Meanwhile the vagina begins to unfold. Its velvety lining, made up of a series of little ripples called rugae (Latin for *wrinkles*), opens like a blossoming flower. The labia part from the pressure of the oncoming head and soon the matted hair and wrinkled scalp of the baby's head are visible in the birth outlet—an exciting landmark.

Another milestone of second stage is touching the baby's head before it is born. The father can remind the mother to do this. When she does, it is often quite exciting.

Toward the end of second stage the baby's head *crowns;* that is, the largest diameter of the head passes through the birth outlet. Crowning is a threshold experience and for many women a moment of panic. The mother may feel stretching, burning sensations, and may even feel as if she is about to split apart. (Of course no one ever does.) But this passes quickly as the head is born.

Shortly after the birth of the head, the shoulders and the rest of the body slip out of the birth canal.

Second stage may last from a few minutes to several hours. The average length is one to two hours.

Third stage follows with a few contractions until the delivery of the placenta—the meaty, disk-shaped organ that was attached to the uterine wall and supplied nutrients to the baby during gestation. Absorbed by her new child, the mother usually pays little attention to this stage. It averages ten to fifteen minutes in length.

Though the purpose of every labor is identical, the birth of a child, every labor is unique. Each has its own individual pattern.

One mother labors for several days with contractions occurring off and on. Another labors and gives birth in a matter of two or three hours. One woman finds labor difficult but not unbearable. Another is overwhelmed with fear and panic. ("It was a terrible ordeal. I never want to go through that again.") Others take labor in stride. ("It wasn't so bad—after all, women all over the world have babies.") Still others experience birth with intense physical and emotional pleasure. ("It was wonderful! I can't wait to have another baby!")

Your labor may be nothing like the labors of women you've read about in books or those you've seen in childbirth films. It may be utterly unlike your friends' labors. It may even be quite different from your own past labor if you've given birth before. But it *can* be a positive, rewarding experience.

The Pain of Labor

Some contractions are painful, others are not. Those that occur toward the end of first stage are usually more painful than early contractions. Some women have less pain than others. A very few report virtually painless labors.

Surrendering to labor and using mental imagery, as discussed later on, will reduce discomfort and help you work *with* the pain. Your partner can also reduce the pain of your labor through giving effective labor support. This is discussed in chapter nine. (In addition, see my book *Sharing Birth: A Father's Guide to Giving Support During Labor.*) But there is nothing you can do to eliminate all the pain, short of using powerful drugs that can interfere with both labor and the baby's health.

However, the pain of labor is unique and is often described as "positive pain." It is *healthy* pain. Each contraction is purposeful. While labor dilates the cervix and opens the gateway so the mother can give birth, it also prepares the baby to be born. The powerful contractions prepare your baby for his first breath. The rhythmically tightening walls of the uterus massage him, stimulating his circulatory system and aiding the expulsion of mucus and fluid from his lungs.

Though it is painful at times, many women find labor extremely fulfilling (which no one would say of a toothache!). Bear in mind that labor is not all pain but encompasses a wide variety of feelings from discomfort to ecstasy.

The Inner Event of Labor

Giving birth involves your whole being: body, mind, and emotions. "Birth is very much a body process," writes Dr. Lewis Mehl in *Birthing Normally*. "It is a process that seems to work best with the woman integrating her consciousness with her body, as a vine climbs a fence row."[2]

Mind and body cannot be separated during labor. We can no more reduce this marvelous process to a series of physical actions than we can reduce lovemaking to mere tension and release in the genitals.

The *inner event of labor* plays a key role in the overall experience of childbearing. The expression *inner event of labor* refers to two basic ideas: (1) the laboring woman's altered state of mind and (2) the sexuality of childbirth. We will discuss each in turn.

The Altered State of Mind of the Laboring Woman

"They say that during the last few hours before birth you lose contact with the outside world," recalls a new mother quoted in Michel Odent's *Birth Reborn*. "This was true of me. I found myself in another universe, on a distant planet, drifting in a sea of sensations."[3]

During early labor the expectant mother may react with a mixture of anxiety and excitement. She may be quite talkative and otherwise act her usual self. But as the cervix continues to dilate during first stage, and later during second stage when the mother bears down, profound psychological changes occur. The laboring woman's mind is altered and passionate emotions are released.

As discussed earlier, the right hemisphere of the brain (associated with intuition, instinct, lovemaking, and labor) becomes more active. The left hemisphere (associated with analysis) becomes less so. As her *heart brain* comes to dominate the scene, the laboring woman becomes more instinctive, more "primitive." She also becomes more introspective. Her focus of concentration narrows. Many mothers forget what they have learned in childbirth classes as a result of their temporary psychological transformation. A woman who plans to watch the birth in a mirror, for example, may be so utterly involved in labor that she forgets to look. She is wholly caught up with the force that will birth her baby.

"It was as if she were in a different world," remarked one father about his partner during late first-stage labor, "traveling in a new dimension as she lay in my arms."

As the mother yields herself more and more to the *inner event of labor,* her partner and her labor are her reality. "If you provide the proper environment," states Dr. Richard B. Stewart of the Birthing Center at Douglas General Hospital in Douglasville, Georgia, "a laboring woman will go into her own psyche and shut out the external world. In fact, if this were done everywhere, every medical institution would have cesarean rates of four or five percent rather than the twenty to thirty percent of most hospitals."

Near the end of labor social inhibitions often melt. Modesty often means little. Many mothers remove their clothing, unconcerned about who sees their naked body or what anyone might think of the passionate sounds they are making. This is particularly common at home or childbearing-center births, where the atmosphere is usually most conducive to a spontaneous response to labor.

"With her vulva wide open and her legs spread apart, it seems as if her entire body is opening up at once," writes Dr. Michel Odent in *Birth Reborn*. "She may even get to the point where she releases her sphincter muscles and empties her rectum. The release of those muscles, and her strong, typical cry, go against the most deeply embedded social behavior. They tell us that the woman in labor has entered the optimum instinctive state of consciousness; in other words, she has achieved the right hormonal balance."[4]

As the force of her labor sweeps through her wave upon wave, the laboring woman radiates her own special beauty. It is as if she is linked by her very roots with the creative power of life.

This uninhibited behavior, far from something to be repressed, should be encouraged. It is normal. *Both* partners should keep this in mind.

Let it happen. Let the *heart brain* take over and labor unfold. As Pascal says so beautifully in his *Pensées*, "The heart has its reasons which reason knows nothing of."

The laboring woman is vulnerable, dependent, and highly sensitive to disturbances in her environment. Anything that affects her emotions or inhibits her self-expression can influence the overall labor process.

Of course the mother wants to know that she is getting fine medical care, is in a safe birthing place, and that all is being done in the best interest of her baby. But she also needs nurturing support and an environment with a positive emotional climate where she can express herself freely during labor and later greet her baby with uninhibited love.

Whatever affects the laboring mind affects the laboring body. Meeting the mother's emotional needs is as essential to a safe, rewarding birth as fulfilling the physical needs. "Whether or not a mother's experience of childbirth is a happy one," writes Bianca Gordon in her article in *The Place of Birth*, "depends not only on the physical care she receives but also on the care for her emotional needs, and on recognition of her as a unique individual."[5]

The laboring woman's unique state of mind makes mental imagery, a means of translating thoughts into images that speak directly to the *heart brain*, a particularly appropriate tool for coping with labor. As one childbirth educator put it, using mental imagery in labor "links the mother up with her instinctive self." It helps her surrender to the *inner event of labor*.

A Peak Experience

"All through labor it was like climbing a mountain—difficult but never more than I could bear. When I got to the summit, I felt like I was at the top of the world and could stoop down and lift the whole earth in my hands. Never in my life have I known such elation. When the baby came I laughed and cried at the same time."

Few events elicit such powerful spiritual feelings as the miracle of reproduction. Lovemaking and birth are often associated with heightened states of consciousness, ecstasy, religious experience, and sometimes a sense of being one with nature or united with all mothers who have ever given birth.

"Giving birth can be a deeply intimate experience for both partners," writes Leni Schwartz in *The World of the Unborn*. "It can be a window to intrinsic patterns of the universe, to cycles of life and death that have existed since the first matter crossed the indefinable line and took the form of living cells. One transcends the ordinary, familiar sense of self to achieve an extraordinary understanding of being one with the cosmos. Women sense their autonomy, at the same time they experience being part of all that is, ever has been, ever will be."[6]

The psychologist Abraham Maslow refers to such a transpersonal state of mind as a "peak experience." "I felt I was one with all mothers," said one mother recalling the moments before birth. Another said: "Waves of creative energy surged through me and I felt part of all forms of life everywhere." Still another remarked, "It was like an orgasm, the greatest orgasm I have ever known."

During our own first birth, my wife Jan bore down as if the whole weight of the earth were upon her. Each new contraction was another burst of cataclysmic energy. "I felt I was being taken over by a power greater than myself," she recalls. "There was nothing I could do about it. It flowed through me like a stream rushing down a mountain. I was absorbed, totally absorbed in the power of birth."

Meanwhile as Jan was pushing I felt I was standing face to face with the power that called life to come forth from the brooding sea. Her vulva opened like a circle in the center of a kaleidoscope. A spot of the baby's head appeared at the end of a little fleshy tunnel. It was just a tiny dot, but for me it was the heart of creation.

Many fathers experience overwhelming ecstatic states during birth. When he first glimpsed the baby's moist head in the birth canal one father said: "I never imagined how intense that moment could be. I was soaring outside myself—in another world."

One needn't seek or expect a spiritual experience in order to birth normally. But couples should be open to the fact that such is often a normal part of labor. After all, birth is nature's greatest miracle.

The Sexuality of Childbirth

From the moment of conception to the time a baby emerges from the uterus slippery and moist to be cradled in mother's arms, childbirth is a sexual process. We can draw striking parallels between lovemaking and uninhibited, unmedicated labor. The following is an expansion of the list Niles Newton includes in *Maternal Emotions:*[7]

- The uterus rhythmically contracts during both intercourse and labor, though the intensity of contractions is far greater in labor.
- The vagina lubricates and opens during both processes.
- Women are usually intensely emotional, vulnerable, and sensitive during both lovemaking and labor.
- An expression of physical exertion appears on a woman's face near orgasm and during childbirth.
- Social inhibitions decrease near sexual climax and toward the end of labor.
- Sensory acuity and awareness of the external environment diminish during both experiences.
- Both orgasm and childbirth are usually followed by a sense of well-being.
- The same hormone, oxytocin, is released during both lovemaking and labor.
- Both lovemaking and labor can be impaired by disturbances in the environment, negative emotions, or inhibitions.
- Lovemaking and labor are both primal functions. Both work best when the judgmental, analytical mind is set aside and the instinctive mind takes over.
- Most important, labor, like lovemaking, is smoothest and most satisfying when one surrenders mind and body to the process.

The fact that labor shares similarities with lovemaking doesn't imply that every moment of labor is pleasurable—though labor can be extraordinarily fulfilling at times. But appreciating the sexual side of labor will help both parents to better relate to the experience.

Damp hair clinging to her perspiring brow, her cheeks flushed with energy, the laboring woman often looks and sounds like a woman at the height of sexual passion. Her breathing may be long and hard. She may moan, sigh and groan, and perhaps make little grunts toward the end of first stage. In second stage, when the urge to give birth sweeps through her, she may moan and grunt as she bears down.

Fathers are sometimes surprised to hear such sounds, and may misinterpret them as expressions of pain. Though groans and sighs may indicate pain, more often than not they are simply the natural, instinctive voice of the laboring woman.

When a laboring woman begins uttering sexual sounds, it often indicates that she has surrendered to labor, that she is attuned to her "primitive" self and is in an optimal state to labor. In effect, her *heart brain* has "taken over."

Making sexual sounds often *helps* the mother better surrender to her sea of sensations. For many laboring women this is a far more effective coping method than fixing the attention on an external object (like a point on the wall or a poster) or trying to control the breathing. In fact, an effective remedy for a mother on the verge of panic is simply to tell her to lower the pitch of her voice. If she is screaming, her partner can tell her to groan or moan instead. If necessary, he can groan with her. The deep, lower-pitched sound often dissolves the fear.

During late labor with their first child in a hospital labor room, one couple spent several contractions on the floor. The mother rested on all fours, a particularly good posture for back pain (back labor) or for a difficult second stage. The father was poised nearby in a similar position. When a contraction began, the mother groaned a long drawn-out "Oooooh!" at the same time revolving her head in a relaxing circle. The father did likewise. At the height of the next contraction both were moaning simultaneously and rather voluminously when their quite conventional obstetrician entered the room. For a few seconds the doctor stood nonplussed, obviously never having seen anything like this before. Then with infinite cool he shrugged his shoulders, exclaimed "Far out!" and left the room.

Though the father may not want to groan with his partner, he can still accept the sounds that she makes and should never discourage her from expressing herself spontaneously during labor (unless she is panic-stricken and screaming).

At one birth when the mother moaned, her husband, meaning well, said: "Don't do that honey! Breathe with me instead." He then demonstrated a panting breath that the couple had learned in childbirth class.

This is poor advice. Telling a laboring woman to stop moaning and instead pant like a dog on a hot summer day can actually *impair* labor. Forcing herself to focus her attention on controlled breathing takes the laboring woman away from her instinctive self.

This doesn't imply that the laboring woman shouldn't use breathing patterns if she wants to. She can learn them in childbirth class and use them *if* she finds them helpful. Some women find controlled breathing the best way to cope with labor. Others do not. The point is that the support person should never suggest that the mother substitute a breathing pattern when she is expressing herself spontaneously.

Of course not all women make sexual sounds or behave in a sexual way when they are otherwise laboring quite normally. It does little good to say, "Moan now, dear!" to the mother who would rather remain quiet or use controlled breathing!

The important thing is that both partners recognize that labor is a sexual experience and that the conditions conducive to satisfying lovemaking are the same conditions that support a fulfilling birth.

Sexuality and Birth: An Inseparable Pair

"Does the woman who has a positive attitude toward her wider sexual role actually have fewer obstetrical and gynecological problems?" asks Niles Newton in *Maternal Emotions*. [8] "Yes!" say many childbirth professionals.

Many midwives and physicians agree that the mother's feelings toward sexual intercourse are related to her experience of childbirth. Women who are comfortable with their bodies and able to express themselves sexually in a natural, uninhibited way are those most likely to take labor in stride.

California nurse midwife June Whitson states: "I have learned to expect that women who are spontaneous about their sexuality, who acknowledge sexual pleasure and are able to talk about it, are probably going to have better birth experiences."

"One could hypothesize," writes Gayle Peterson in *Birthing Normally*, "that in sexually repressed cultures, a prolonged and painful labor may be symptomatic of the fight against the sexuality of the experience. The greater the fight, the greater the increase in stress. Likewise, the more stress experienced around the conflict of sexuality, during birth, the greater the occurrence of complication due to the accumulation of stress."[9]

In fact, a positive attitude toward sexuality is important even for those attending the birth on a professional level. The authors Jensen, Benson, and Bobak state in the text *Maternity Care: The Nurse and the Family*, "The first task of the maternity nurse is to come to terms with her own sexuality."[10] More and more professionals realize that comfort with their own sexuality is indispensable in effectively helping laboring women.

Labor and birth take place within the sexual organs. Respect and admiration for our sexual anatomy and sexual feelings enhance a healthy birthing attitude. The better both parents feel about sexuality, the more likely they will be able to participate wholeheartedly in the birth experience.

Sexual repression, on the other hand, can also be carried into the birthing room, and a sexually inhibited woman is likely to have a more difficult time surrendering to the powerful sensations of labor.

Pregnancy is a good time to appreciate the sexual organs and the almost unbelievable changes they experience. Touch and loving communication between partners is also especially important during pregnancy's sensitive months.

Learning about the Sexuality of Childbirth

Appreciating the sexuality of childbirth is a long step toward understanding labor. If possible, attend classes and view films that convey the sexual dimensions of childbearing. Some films show women expressing themselves spontaneously. These give a far better picture of the sensuality of childbearing than do films depicting a laboring woman wearing a hospital johnnie and exhibiting a remarkable and unrealistic degree of self-control while her partner stands by holding her hand and coaching her with breathing. A far more appropriate place for the father is lying or sitting on the bed, embracing and caressing her—or remaining at her side if she is up walking.

With an appreciation for the sexuality of childbirth the mother can better surrender to labor. She can give herself to the experience without fear. The father acquainted with birth's sexual side is prepared to accept his partner's perhaps irrational behavior, seeing her changes as positive signs rather than as part of a frightening experience he doesn't understand. Most important, he is better able to give labor support that is appropriate to the mother's experience. For example, caressing his partner and sharing his love are at times far more effective than coaching her with breathing patterns. In fact, loving and even sexual contact can actually speed up labor. Elisabeth Bing's observation in *Making Love During Pregnancy* is well known today: "Stimulation of the breasts and other erogenous zones releases hormones that seem to speed up the pace of labor."[11]

Many childbirth professionals understand and appreciate the primal beauty and distinctly sexual behavior of the laboring woman. But bear in mind that many do not. This is evidenced by the clinical environment in which some American women are expected to labor normally. Routine procedures such as perineal

shaving and replacing personal apparel with hospital clothing—
procedures that bear more the character of ritual than science—
render the expectant mother an almost *asexual* being. Fortunately, such routines are falling by the wayside; obstetrics is
changing. Meanwhile, the expectant parents must take responsibility to plan their birth wisely, taking the sexual nature of the
experience into consideration.

On the other side of the coin, some laboring women are more
comfortable if they do not view birth as a sexual event. The
thought of sexuality makes them more tense. In this case, covering the legs with drapes may actually make the laboring woman
more comfortable and better able to surrender to labor. The
mother should do whatever best reduces her tension and inhibitions.

Making Your Labor Work for You: Surrendering

The *inner event of labor* is largely the foundation for the steps
in this book. As mentioned previously, *whatever affects the laboring
mind affects the laboring body*. Each step in *Mind Over Labor* re-
volves around the fact that labor triggers an altered state of mind
and that labor is a sexual process.

Everything you do to prepare for labor, from making birth
plans to hiring a caregiver to assist you during childbirth, should
be done with the *inner event of labor* in mind. When you make
birth plans take into consideration the laboring woman's altered
state of mind and the sexuality of the experience. If your birth
plans and your basic attitude toward birth reflect an appreciation
for labor's inner event, you will be sure to create the conditions
for labor to unfold smoothly.

"Sometimes labor is hard and sometimes it is painful," said
one new mother. "But when you learn to trust your body, you
know you can do it. The secret is letting go and letting your
body work for you. It is welcoming each contraction; each one
is a step closer to seeing your baby."

The more you are able to yield to the *inner event of labor* and to your unfamiliar bodily sensations, to let go and give yourself to the experience, the better your chance of an efficient labor. "Think of a time when you really wanted to open for your lover," one childbirth educator tells her clients. "How you felt all open and vulnerable, yet so willing. This is how you should open for your baby."

Anxiety and the desire to control labor can hinder it. For example, a mother's labor slows down. Perhaps someone then makes a comment about her "slow labor." This makes her nervous and she may worry about having a cesarean. She wants her body to work for her. But there seems to be nothing she can do. Like trying to have an orgasm, the harder one tries, the more elusive it seems. The best thing to do is stop trying: Surrender to the process.

One purpose of using mental imagery in labor is to help you say yes to labor, to flow with the experience rather than try to control it. In his excellent guided-imagery tape "Great Expectations," Dr. Emmett Miller reminds the laboring woman, "You don't have to lead, you can follow, observing, letting your body do it, letting your body guide you through this wonderful process of birth."[12]

Surrender is the key. It will make you a partner rather than an adversary of the life-creating force.

∾ CHAPTER THREE

Developing a Positive Image of Birth:
THE SECOND STEP

> We shall not cease from exploration
> And the end of all our exploring
> Will be to arrive where we started
> And know the place for the first time.
> —T. S. Eliot

"What happens at birth," asserts Lester Hazell, the former president of the International Childbirth Education Association (ICEA), "tends to be guided by our belief system about birth."

A positive image of birth is the cornerstone of a safe, happy birth experience. If you believe your body is meant to give birth efficiently, naturally, and without complications and that birth is a joyful event, you are more than halfway to a safe, natural birth. Positive beliefs and attitudes contribute to a happy birth experience, enabling the mother to labor more efficiently and to open for her baby with less effort.

The way you view birth will shape your overall childbearing experience, your birth plans, your labor, and the period after the baby is born.

Beliefs regulate actions. Many people believe, for example, that birth is a medical crisis and that the highly technological medical center is the safest place to give birth. The mother who thinks this way will choose such an environment. She plans her birth according to her beliefs.

Beliefs influence labor. According to Dr. Emmett Miller, images that produce stress and fear tend to cause tension of the musculature and imbalances in both blood flow and hormone secretion, which can inhibit labor. The mother can hold her labor back unconsciously if she is not ready for her baby to be born or if she mistrusts her body.

In *Silent Knife*, the classic of cesarean prevention, Nancy Wainer Cohen and Lois Estner write: "Your beliefs about yourself, your body, your baby, your life, your power, will influence your birth. If you see your body as a well-functioning trusted partner in birth, your experience will be different from that of someone who is confused, self-conscious, and insecure about her body. Your mind will influence your body. . . . The fact that our beliefs, our thoughts about ourselves, affect our births helps to explain, for example, why many women with an 'inadequate' or questionable pelvis give birth to 8, 9 or 10 pound infants, while other women with totally adequate pelves have difficulty or are unable to deliver their 6½ to 7 pound babies."[1]

Your image of birth will even influence whether or not you have a cesarean section. Though cesarean surgery can be a life-saving operation in the face of grave medical complications, the vast majority of cesareans, many childbirth professionals agree, are avoidable. The reason for America's 20 percent cesarean rate lies not so much in physical causes (though these certainly play a role) as in beliefs and attitudes about birth. In fact, nothing so clearly reveals the influence of negative attitudes on human birth as does our outrageous cesarean rate.

Underlying the almost casual acceptance of cesarean surgery is a basic mistrust of the body and of nature. Surgical delivery is often the final symptom of the myth that medically managed labor is better than natural labor, or that a woman can't give birth to a healthy baby without the help of technological intervention.

Such myths, held by many childbirth professionals and parents alike, shatter the most precious experience of hundreds of thousands of women every year.

Negative beliefs, of course, are not solely responsible for unnecessary cesareans. Other factors such as the birthing environment, the caregiver, how the caregiver manages labor and delivery, and the mother's labor support influence whether she births surgically or normally.

Nevertheless, beliefs can contribute to a cesarean more than most women realize. Cohen and Estner have found that a high number of cesarean mothers hold beliefs that are *not* conducive to normal birth. Many, for example, have little confidence in their bodies and in the birth process and hold the belief that birth is unsafe or a medical event. It is essential to let go of such beliefs and replace them with positive images, beliefs, and attitudes.

Your image of birth may also affect your postpartum recovery period. The birthing environment you choose, for example, will influence the quality of time you and your partner can spend with the baby immediately after birth. This, in turn, will greatly influence your postpartum feelings and perhaps whether or not you experience postpartum depression. (This subject is discussed further in chapter ten.)

Letting Go of Myths

Childbirth in America is like a Picasso painting. What you see doesn't make a lot of sense at first. For example, many people picture birth with IVs, electronic fetal monitors, hideous hospital johnnies fully open at the back, sterile delivery rooms, mothers birthing in the flat-on-the-back position with legs in stirrups as helpless as upside-down turtles, masked attendants milling about, and so forth. Not only is the medical value of such things questionable, but they actually rob an expectant mother of her self-confidence and draw a curtain between her and the wonderful experience birth can be. That many perfectly healthy women actually give birth this way and that some consider this normal is an utter absurdity.

Fortunately this is changing and a saner view of birth is emerging. Yet a body of myths still clings to childbirth. Many expectant parents and childbirth professionals approach birth as if they believe that childbirth is an illness or somehow abnormal; that birth is unsafe for mother and baby; that a woman's body is incompetent and will not function properly without medical intervention and technological aid; and that a large percentage of women are unable to birth naturally.

These myths have become so ingrained in our thinking that they pervade the mental picture of labor and actually shape the birth experience of many women. They are reinforced by some hospitals and childbirth professionals.

A vague belief in women's incompetence is woven into our overall picture of childbirth like an insidious thread—a thread that all but ties a noose around mothers' necks when they enter the hospital. Will I be unable to birth normally? Will there be complications? Will I need a cesarean? Is my pelvis adequate? One or all of these fears haunt most expectant mothers.

A common, none too pleasant expression circulates among computer programmers: "Garbage in, garbage out" (sometimes abbreviated GIGO). Your mind is not a computer and your body is not a machine. But the rough comparison holds: If you "program" your mind with negative beliefs and attitudes, you are likely to have a negative outcome.

Childbirth myths commonly held in our culture need not influence you. Ask yourself what you believe about birth. Explore your beliefs. If you identify a myth in yourself that might interfere with normal birthing, release it. Replace it with a positive view such as that outlined in the next section.

The Five Essentials of a Positive, Healthy View of Birth

Next to eating nutritiously, developing a positive attitude about birth is probably the most important step an expectant mother can take toward ensuring a safe, fulfilling birth. Examining one's beliefs and cultivating a positive attitude might not be necessary if our culture didn't harbor myths or if the medical profession had a less peculiar attitude about childbirth. But as it is, the expectant parents must take responsibility for their own views.

The expectant father too should cultivate a positive view. If he is present during labor, his attitude will influence his partner's labor. If he believes her body is capable of birthing naturally, he will be able to give more effective support than if he views birth as a clinical procedure.

Following are the essentials of a positive birth image:

Birth is a natural process, not a medical event. Trusting the body to birth naturally is a long step toward a safe, rewarding birth. Faith that the power of nature will fulfill its purpose in the life-creating miracle is worth a dozen childbirth classes.

It may sound absurd to remind a mother that birth is natural. Yet this seemingly obvious fact needs to be reinforced in a country with a 20 percent cesarean rate. In our society labor is viewed largely within a medical frame of reference. The fact that birth most often takes place in a hospital setting prevents us from seeing birth as a natural part of our lives.

Today, with our emphasis on medical technology, we often lose sight of the birth process itself. It is almost as if we forget that it is the mother who gives birth, not the attendants around her. Good prenatal care and the assistance of a competent care-giver during labor are important for a healthy mother and baby. But this doesn't mean that birth is a medical event.

The expression "natural childbirth" is used in a variety of contexts to describe everything short of major abdominal surgery.

In some hospitals, although the mother is barely conscious during the birth of her child, she is said to have birthed naturally whether or not she has had an episiotomy (surgical incision to enlarge the birth outlet), medication, or even epidural anesthesia. However, true natural birth refers to more than vaginal delivery in whatever form; it means birthing without any unnecessary intervention, as nature designed.

Appreciating that birth is a natural event doesn't necessarily mean that the mother is committed to laboring and giving birth with no medication (though this is usually safer for her and her child). Rather it implies that the mother believes that birth is not a medical but a natural physiologic process like conception.

Birth is a normal process, not an illness. The corollary to the idea that birth is natural is that giving birth is *normal,* another seemingly obvious statement.

Labor is a physiologic function which in most cases occurs without complications. Of course, no one actually thinks that childbearing is an illness. But many parents and childbirth professionals *act as if it were.*

Birth is a time of psychological stress for the entire family simply because it is such a life-altering event. However, as Gayle Peterson points out in *Birthing Normally,* "Contrary to the belief that birth is traumatic, my experience with women birthing their babies has led me to a view of birth as a healthy stress."[2]

It is essential to make a place in the heart for normal birth so that it can become a reality. This doesn't mean that the mother shouldn't give birth in a hospital if that is where she feels most comfortable. It means that wherever she plans to birth, she should release the myth that the laboring woman is some sort of invalid and replace it with an image of health and beauty. This is no exercise in self-deception. The laboring woman *is* radiantly healthy—she is at the height of her creative power.

Birth is a social event. The beginning of a family, birth is the most significant social event in the lives of most couples. Labor is an initiation into a new mode of being. As labor ushers you and your partner across the one-way bridge to parenthood, this dramatic passage rite initiates the baby into life outside the womb.

Birth is a celebration of life. Think of your birth as you would your wedding. Dr. Philip Sumner of Manchester, Connecticut, a pioneer in the development of the birthing room, agrees: "childbirth should be like a wedding: just as personal and just as special."[3] Of course, the two situations are quite different. However, they are both life-altering social events for you and your partner. Viewing birth as you would your wedding gives you a fresh perspective of the childbearing miracle and will help you make plans conducive to normal birth. If you plan your birth as carefully as most couples plan their wedding, you will avoid much disappointment.

You are the center of the childbearing drama. It is your birth, your baby, your strength and power that will bring the baby into the world.

I'm often amazed to hear new mothers say such things as, "The hospital allowed my mother to remain with us during delivery," or "The doctor let me touch my baby as she was born" (as if being allowed to touch one's baby were an extraordinary thing!). You *choose* the place where you will give birth. You *invite* your caregiver to attend and pay a fee for the caregiver's services. You are the employer, the boss. Don't lose sight of this.

When you go into labor, it is *your* day, not the hospital's or the caregiver's. They are there to serve you, not to take over your experience. You and your partner alone have the *right* and the *responsibility* to make decisions regarding the circumstances of your birth, just as you would about any other important occasion of life.

This includes such things as what you will do in labor (everything from the use of medical intervention to what you will eat, drink, wear, and whether you will go out for a walk), who will attend your birth (just you and your partner, or family and friends), how much time you will spend with the baby after birth, and so on. To whatever degree possible, all decisions must remain your own.

You are responsible for making wise choices. Taking responsibility for your birth goes hand in hand with seeing yourself as the center of the childbearing drama. This means accepting that it is up to you to plan your birth wisely, to create the optimal environment to begin your family, and to invite those who will assist you carefully.

Of course the mother wants to do what is in the best interest of her baby. But this doesn't mean throwing oneself into a caregiver's hands or choosing the hospital nearest home. Since there are so many varied options available, the consumer of obstetrical care must take active responsibility to explore options and make sensible choices.

Understanding the *inner event of labor* and keeping these five essentials in mind will help you make wise choices.

Elements That Influence Your Birth

A process of both physical and psychological transformation, childbirth is always a life-altering occasion. But giving birth is not an isolated event. It is influenced by a woman's entire history. All the mother's feelings, apprehensions, joys, and doubts about her body, pregnancy, and parenthood play a part in her experience of labor.

Healthy beliefs and attitudes support a positive birth experience like the nutrients in the soil nourish a thriving garden. By getting familiar with your beliefs you are "testing the soil." You discover whether or not what you believe is conducive to natural birth. If not, you can reshape your views and replace negative with positive attitudes.

Your attitudes about birth may be hazy and indistinct, perhaps even unconscious, but they can still influence your labor. "Childbearing sets off many emotionally charged memories in our mental computer banks, memories that might otherwise remain unconscious and out of awareness," states Claudia Panuthos in *Transformation Through Birth.* "Childbearing is a time of great change, physically and emotionally. Because it is such a transitional period, it is an opportune time for women to rethink their former beliefs, values and attitudes and to replace any historical mental systems that are not devoted to total well-being with new mental attitudes that are."[4]

As stated earlier, whatever affects the *inner event of labor* affects labor's physiology. Following are the most common psychological factors that can impair labor:

- An environment unsuitable for spontaneous self-expression
- A caregiver, nurse, or other person in the environment with whom you are uncomfortable
- Excessive fear
- Strong beliefs that are not conducive to normal birth
- Unresolved emotional conflicts about becoming a parent
- An emotional conflict or tension between you and your partner
- Excessive self-consciousness and/or anxiety about performing in a certain way during labor
- Insecurity about your body
- Excessive modesty
- Sexual repression

Rahima Baldwin, author of *Special Delivery,* says that factors such as those listed above can lead to what she calls psychological dystocia (*dystocia* means impaired labor).[5] This doesn't imply that every woman who has one or more of the above will have a terrible labor. They are simply emotional factors that *may* impair labor. One benefit of the method in this book is eliminating such factors whenever possible and living as best you can with those you are unable to change.

Meanwhile, pay special attention to the other steps in *Mind Over Labor*. As Dr. Michel Odent says in *Birth Reborn*, "We can't miraculously erase a woman's preconceptions and past experiences, but we can create an atmosphere that will encourage women and their partners to approach birth differently."[6]

Examine your feelings. It isn't necessary to have the same outlook as someone you know or have read about who has had a positive birth experience. The main thing is greeting birth positively and in your own way.

Feelings about Parenthood

Confronting your feelings about impending parenthood during pregnancy is a vital part of childbirth preparation. This will enable you to greet your labor more positively, make a smoother transition to your new life after the baby is born, and reduce the chance of postpartum blues.

If she doesn't feel she is ready to give birth, the mother may hold back psychologically. "If the marital relationship is in question, or finances are a serious problem," write Nancy Cohen and Lois Estner in *Silent Knife*, "a mother's instinct to keep her baby inside may conflict with the baby's readiness to labor. Half-way up the mountain, the climb seems too high and the fall too steep."[7]

One mother, who had been in labor for twenty hours, failed to progress (her cervix didn't dilate). Her midwife felt this was the result of emotional factors. Labor had begun before the mother's due date and she wasn't prepared for the baby. The midwife suggested that the mother relax and try to make whatever emotional adjustments were necessary. The mother fell asleep. When she awoke, her contractions were strong and the baby was born shortly.

Discuss your feelings about parenthood—both negative and positive—with your partner. Don't expect to create an unconditionally positive view toward having a baby. Nearly all expectant parents have reservations. Is it really the right time? Will

I be a good mother? father? How are we going to afford to feed another mouth? Will our relationship ever be the same? How will our lives change? Most every expectant mother and father ask themselves such questions.

Accept your ambivalent feelings as normal. The important thing is that there be no overwhelming hindrances—and that you *know* what you feel. Strong emotional conflicts should be resolved before labor whenever possible.

Using mental imagery to confront feelings and help resolve potential conflicts about parenthood is discussed in chapter six.

Your Mother, Other Relatives, and Friends

What you have learned from close relatives and friends helps shape your view of birth. What have you been told to expect? What can you remember about the births of brothers and sisters? Family religious beliefs may also affect the way an expectant mother feels about sexuality and childbirth.

Your relationship with your mother influences the way you birth and, of course, mother your own child. Most women experience intense thoughts and feelings about their mothers during pregnancy; many relive and reevaluate their relationship.

You might ask your mother what her birth experience was like, whether or not she breastfed and why. Talking about this may bring you and your mother closer; she may reexperience her childbearing and you may discover what helped shape your present attitudes.

Your mother's experience need not be a model for your own. Remember that many women were unconscious during delivery not so long ago. Much has changed since the era of what Dr. Robert Bradley calls "knock 'em out, drag 'em out obstetrics."

If your mother had a negative birth experience, share it with her, empathize, but be aware that you don't have to repeat it. Few complications run in the family.

If friends have had less than positive birth experiences, be aware that this has no bearing on your own birth. You can make entirely different plans, choose a different caregiver or birthing place, and above all, shape your attitudes so that they will contribute to a safe, happy birth.

Releasing Negative Feelings about Prior Births

Perhaps the birth you are now anticipating and preparing for is not your first. A previous birth may not have turned out as you would have liked. If so, it is natural to harbor negative feelings about childbirth. Some women feel they have failed if things didn't happen the way they expected. Many men feel they failed to give their partners adequate support during pregnancy, labor, or afterward. Though there is no such thing as failure in childbirth, there is disappointment, hurt, resentment, anger, and grief.

Your grief may be for anything from unfulfilled expectations to loss of a child. You may feel cheated if your needs and wishes in labor were not respected or if you had to have an unexpected cesarean.

If your feelings about a past birth haven't yet been resolved, now is the time to examine, confront, and release them. Failure to do so can give them exaggerated importance and influence your present birth.

Many women who are upset over thwarted expectations receive little support from their health caregiver, relatives, and friends, who may not understand and may even feel that there's nothing to be upset about as long as one has a healthy baby.

Discuss your feelings with your partner, a friend, or a professional counselor if necessary. Some counselors specialize in birth-related problems.

Anger at a physician or nurse who attended your birth may sometimes be appropriate. Perhaps you can channel that energy into helping reshape the obstetrical system. Diana Korte and Roberta Scaer in *A Good Birth, A Safe Birth* suggest that those who have been the victims of medical intervention or an insensitive hospital system become change makers themselves.[8]

In *Silent Knife* Nancy Cohen and Lois Estner recommend using mental imagery to facilitate emotional healing if the mother and baby have been separated after a cesarean birth. Their suggestions can be adapted to other situations as well. They advise that one imagine the moments after delivery and recreate the scene in the mind's eye. For example, the mother can imagine she is holding her baby close and telling the baby "all that she didn't have the chance to say before he was taken from her."[9]

A mother who tried this imagery later told her eight-year-old daughter of her sad and lonely feelings. "It was a very special moment," Cohen and Estner write, quoting the mother.

The authors also suggest another healing image: "A woman who has been separated from her baby can also imagine that before her infant is taken from her, she is giving him a special gift. This gift should symbolize all the love she has for her baby. She can imagine that her baby reaches out, takes the gift, and cuddles it close to his heart."[10]

This sort of imagery and the feelings it evokes can help free one of the burden of negative emotion and bring about true healing.

A final important step in resolving conflicts about past births is to forgive and release those involved. Harboring resentment will make emotional healing more difficult. You can try picturing the person in your mind's eye and saying, "I fully and freely forgive and release you. I am free and you are free."

If you can't bring yourself to forgive a particular person, Elsye Birkinshaw suggests (in her book *Think Slim—Be Slim*) asking God to forgive that person in your name.[11] Above all, forgive yourself.

Now is the time to turn your attention to this birth, to make the birth for which you are now preparing the kind of experience you really want.

A significant emotional conflict about parenthood, a past birth, or sexuality and childbirth in general can inhibit normal birth.

If you feel you have such a conflict and have difficulty resolving it on your own, don't hesitate to seek counseling.

Additional aids to cultivating a positive view of birth include:

- Taking time to appreciate the body and the miracle it is working.
- Choosing a caregiver with a positive birth attitude (discussed in chapter eight).
- Attending childbirth classes that support natural childbirth and inspire confidence in *both* partners (discussed in chapter six).
- Reading books that discuss natural childbirth in a positive light (see the references at the end of this book).
- Using supportive statements such as those on pages 73–74 when you practice relaxation and imagery.

Every step you take to develop a positive birth image is a step closer to a safe, rewarding childbearing experience. Bear in mind, however, that you may not be able to alter all your views and feelings. After all, they have been acquired over a lifetime and will probably not change overnight. For now the important thing is keeping an open mind.

Dr. David Stewart, medical statistician and executive director of NAPSAC International (the InterNational Association for Parents and Professionals for Safe Alternatives in Childbirth), states: "Although my wife, Lee, felt some anxiety from time to time in pregnancy, the closer it came to the time for labor, the less fear she felt. During labor she felt no fear at all. This was to a great extent the result of consciously working to clear her mind of all negativity and doubt as well as sending positive and loving thoughts to her unborn child throughout pregnancy. The result was a fear-free, complication-free birth in five pregnancies out of five. Though we coupled our mental and spiritual efforts with excellent nutrition and physical exercise, the fundamental factor in our bearing healthy babies was not of the body, but of the mind."

Allow yourself to feel enthusiastic about giving birth. "Pessimists may comment that one should not aspire to natural childbirth in case complications develop," writes Elizabeth Noble in *Childbirth With Insight*. "This is like saying one shouldn't bond with the baby in case it dies, or one shouldn't fall in love in case one gets hurt. Such timidity and anti-life sentiments lead to self-fulfilling prophecies and deny the human potential to respond to the unexpected."[12]

✑ CHAPTER FOUR

Relaxing Mind and Body:
THE THIRD STEP

The relaxation exercises in this chapter will (1) enable you to make the most effective use of the mental imagery exercises in the chapters ahead (mental imagery works best when mind and body are relaxed), and (2) give you a far greater ability to relax in labor, thereby reducing the fear, pain, and in some cases even the length of labor.

Relaxation is the key to opening the way for your baby in the shortest, least uncomfortable way. A woman in average physical condition who can relax will almost certainly have a less stressful labor than the most athletic woman who is tense.

Fear-Tension-Pain

As already discussed, fear can cause the cervix to remain resistant to dilation, thereby causing a longer, more painful labor. Dr. Grantly Dick-Read, a pioneer in the field of natural childbirth and the author of *Childbirth Without Fear*, recalls an incident that illustrates how fear and tension affect labor. Upon examining a laboring woman he found her cervix loose and opening wide. A few more labor contractions should have expanded it sufficiently to allow the baby to pass. But when the next contraction occurred, the mother reacted with intense fear, clutching the nurse around the waist and seizing the pillow in an agonized expression of pain. *Her cervix tightened to a size no bigger than a quarter!*[1]

This is one way that tension impairs labor. The nervous woman is often the slowest to dilate. A tense woman—a tense cervix. A tense cervix—a longer labor.

Dr. Read, writing in the 1930s, insisted that fear is the most significant cause of a painful and overly long labor. Fear triggers what he called the "fear-tension-pain cycle": A contraction begins. The laboring woman reacts with fear. She tenses. Her tension causes pain. This in turn increases her fear, which leads to greater tension, and so on as the cycle spirals.

One cannot attribute all of labor's discomfort to fear and tension. Labor is uncomfortable for most women no matter how relaxed they are. But fear and tension can increase pain.

Fear and tension interfere with what Dr. Read called "the neuromuscular harmony of labor."[2] The fight-or-flight state of mind prevents the mother from surrendering to both the physical sensations and the *inner event of labor.*

"The secret of rapid opening of the outlet of the uterus," Dr. Read writes, "is to allow the skeletal muscles to become limp and thus let the uterus work by itself."[3] The soft and stretchable cervix generally opens without resistance in a relaxed mother, while in a tense woman it can remain closed even through increasingly difficult contractions.

"My labor was difficult because I was so afraid," said Lisa, recalling the birth of her first child. "I knew I was holding back. But with the next few contractions the midwife helped me relax by telling me to imagine myself floating up over ocean waves and to think of getting ready to greet my baby. The difference was amazing. Labor was still a struggle. But I felt that I was cooperating, not fighting with it. Things started to pick up." (The imagery of floating on the waves, which many find quite effective, is in chapter six.)

When a contraction begins, the frightened woman tends to

draw in her abdomen and hold her breath. The tense abdominal muscles press against the sensitive contracting uterus, causing pain. "Fear also affects the circulation of the blood to and from the uterus," Dr. Read points out, "for persisting tension of the uterine musculature prevents complete relaxation between contractions. The great blood sinuses of the uterus are deprived of full expansion and the venous blood, replete with metabolites, or waste products of muscular action, are unable to discard their contents as freely as they should."[4] Restricted circulation increases muscle pain. The uterus becomes hypersensitive, sometimes even painful to a light touch.

In addition, restricted circulation deprives the baby of an adequate supply of fresh oxygen. Severe tension may lead to fetal distress, prompting a cesarean section.

Excessive tension may also increase the discomfort and length of the bearing-down (or pushing) process—though for many women this is the least uncomfortable (and sometimes quite an enjoyable) part of labor. Tension can shut the outlet of the birth canal. The tense woman holds back as the baby descends, rather than yielding to labor and allowing the birth outlet to open. The pelvic floor musculature tightens; the vaginal sphincter (the ringlike muscle that controls the vaginal opening) constricts; the perineum (area between the vagina and anus) remains rigid.

Meanwhile the uterus works harder in an effort to birth the baby through a tight and resistant birth canal. It is like pulling a door open with one hand and pushing it closed with the other. As a result, the chances of lacerations and injury to maternal tissue, abnormal discomfort, and a prolonged labor are increased.

On the other hand, if the muscles of the birth canal are relaxed and yielding, giving birth is less uncomfortable. It takes less time for the baby to ease through the stretchable birth outlet. You will also have a better chance of birthing without tearing, and if you don't tear you will be considerably more comfortable during the postpartum period. Finally, by being relaxed you will have more energy for the exciting moments after your baby is born.

Dr. Read's colleagues were astounded that many women he attended didn't seem to suffer despite the fact that no medication was used. A few actually wondered if he had mystical powers. But it wasn't magic that helped his patients birth naturally. It was his emphasis on relaxation and on a positive view of birth. His teaching inspired confidence and encouraged mothers to trust their bodies and the process of labor. His patients were able to break the cycle of fear-tension-pain.

You also can break this vicious cycle. The relaxation exercises in this chapter and the mental imagery exercises ahead will show you how.

BENEFITS OF RELAXATION IN LABOR

- Interrupts the fear-tension-pain cycle
- Decreases discomfort
- May shorten labor
- Gives more energy for second and third stages
- Helps avoid tearing
- Reduces fatigue during and after birth

About Fear

"I'm afraid."

It is the universal comment. Virtually all women approach labor feeling vulnerable. All have doubts and anxieties about giving birth. Nearly every pregnant woman—however excited about seeing her baby—is afraid of labor, especially if it is her first birth and labor is an unknown experience.

Though you will be able to reduce the fear and tension of labor considerably with relaxation and mental imagery, don't expect to eliminate *all* the fear. It is natural to be apprehensive about labor. Even if you have read dozens of books on the subject, that still doesn't tell you what labor will be like for you.

Eliminating all the fear from birth is unnecessary. But since uncontrolled fear can increase labor's discomfort, cause prolonged labor, and heighten the possibility of complications, reducing *excessive* fear is vital. You can do this with steps 1, 2, 3, and 4: understanding labor, developing a positive view of birth, mastering relaxation, and using mental imagery.

Practicing Mind/Body Relaxation

The kind of relaxation you should practice to reduce pain and shorten labor involves more than just sitting back and watching TV, reading a good novel, or having a drink before dinner to "unwind." It requires eliminating all unnecessary mental and physical tension.

Most people living in today's fast-paced society have to practice relaxation in order to master it. But everyone can learn to relax. Practicing regularly (two or three days a week) in the third trimester of pregnancy will teach your body the feeling of muscular release so that by the time labor begins, relaxation will be second nature.

Here are some guidelines:

- Practice relaxation in a place where you won't be disturbed—a quiet room with soft lighting. Wear loose comfortable clothing and take off your shoes. If you wear glasses, remove them. The bladder should be emptied before you begin so you will not be interrupted.
- Practice at the same time each day, if possible, so that preparing for labor will take on a regular pattern—and so you won't forget to practice! An especially good time is following aerobic exercise (hiking, bicycling, swimming, etc.), yoga, or exercises specifically designed for pregnant women. However, any time you practice will be beneficial.
- Practice with your partner, if possible. This will better pre-

pare you to work together in labor. By following the directions on pages 61–62 your partner can learn to check your relaxation, recognize signs of tension, and give valuable feedback.

You both can read through the instructions and then do the exercise together. Or your partner (or a friend) can read the instructions to you. The person reading aloud should do so in a soft, gentle voice, pausing between each step to allow you time to complete it.

• Try an audio cassette tape. This is an effective and, some will find, easier way to learn relaxation than by reading through instructions and then following them. The cassette "Letting Go of Stress" by Emmett Miller, M.D., includes "Progressive Relaxation" (pages 53–55), an autogenic relaxation exercise similar to that on pages 56–57, and two additional exercises. You can use "Letting Go of Stress" either in conjunction with the other exercises in this chapter or in place of them. To order it, see the reference section at the end of this book.

• Practice relaxation in any comfortable position. Many people find lying on the back most effective when first learning to relax. Hatha yoga technique recommends lying flat with arms slightly away from the sides, fingers comfortably curled, and legs slightly apart.

You can vary this position by using pillows wherever comfortable: under your head, knees, elbows, and so forth.

Back-lying can impede circulation in late pregnancy. *Don't lie on your back if it makes you feel dizzy or uncomfortable. Always avoid back-lying in labor. In this position the uterus puts pressure on major blood vessels and reduces the flow of blood to the placenta.*

Other relaxation positions for late pregnancy include:

—Semi-reclining with head and shoulders supported by pillows, knees bent and resting on cushions

—Side-lying with head and shoulders resting on pillows

and a pillow between the knees
    —Sitting on a well-supported surface such as a large easy chair or a bean-bag chair
- Raise yourself up slowly when you finish your relaxation exercise to avoid dizziness or lightheadedness.

Note: Some of the exercises may seem quite lengthy as you read through them, particularly Progressive Relaxation and Circulating the Life Breath. But there is much repetition and the instructions are easily learned.

You are bound to be more deeply relaxed while practicing at home than when you are experiencing the unfamiliar sensations of labor in a hospital or childbearing center. But learning total mind/body relaxation now will make it easier for you to relax sufficiently when the drama of labor begins.

It is not necessary to meet every contraction in labor with total muscular release. Sitting, lying, or standing about like a limp noodle during labor is both unnatural and unnecessary. The goal of practicing relaxation is to eliminate *excessive* tension and to be more able to surrender to the childbearing process.

Methods of Mind/Body Relaxation

Following are several methods of achieving a relaxed state of body and mind. Experiment to find which ones appeal to you and practice those that you find most effective.

Progressive Relaxation

If at first you have difficulty releasing muscular tension (many people do), this exercise will help. Step by step you tense and release muscle groups until you achieve complete physical relaxation. Progressive relaxation is an excellent way to learn complete muscular release. (The relaxation method owes its name to the book *Progressive Relaxation* by Edmund Jacobson).[5]

Releasing muscular tension may take some concentration at first. But it will soon become easier and more natural. (Don't be intimidated by this exercise. Though it is long, the wording is repetitious and the exercise very effective.)

Get into a comfortable position.

Close your eyes.

Take a few slow, deep breaths in through the nose, exhaling through slightly parted lips.

As you begin to relax, let your breathing become just a little deeper and a little slower without straining in any way.

Now tighten the muscles of your left arm and hand, clenching your fist. Hold for a few seconds.

Feel the tension.

Release, letting your arm and hand go limp.

Feel the relaxation.

Tighten the muscles of your right arm and hand, clenching your fist. Hold for a few seconds.

Feel the tension.

Release, letting your arm and hand go limp.

Feel the relaxation.

For the next few minutes, each time you tense a muscle group, feel the tension. Each time you release, take a few seconds to feel the relaxation.

Tighten the muscles of your left leg and foot, curling the toes.

Release, letting your leg and foot go limp.

Tighten the muscles of your right leg and foot, curling the toes.

Release, letting your leg and foot go limp.

Squeeze your buttocks together tightly.

Release.

Draw up the muscles of the pelvic floor (as if you were trying to hold back from urinating).

Release.

Tighten your abdominal muscles, drawing in your belly as if you were trying to touch your backbone with your abdominal wall.

Release. Feel your abdomen relax completely.

Arch your back slightly.

Release, letting the muscles of your back sink into the surface on which you are lying or sitting.

Tighten your shoulders by pushing them back as if you were trying to make the shoulder blades touch one another.

Release, letting the shoulders fall limp.

Tighten the muscles of your neck by arching the neck slightly as if you were trying to look up.

Release, letting your neck go limp.

Clench your teeth together, tightening the muscles of your jaw.

Release.

Squint your eyes.

Release, letting the eyelids fall heavy.

Furrow your brow as if you were worried about something.

Release, letting the space between the eyes feel as if it were getting wider.

Now take a few deep breaths, letting your breathing become a little slower, a little deeper than usual, without straining in any way.

Let your awareness travel through your entire body from head to toe, releasing any additional tension you may find on the out-breath.

Enjoy the feeling of being relaxed, letting yourself know that each time you do this exercise, it will be a little easier.

When you are ready, open your eyes and gently stretch.

Using Suggestion

Once you know the feeling of total body relaxation, you can get in a comfortable position and tell yourself to relax. Go over the entire body one area at a time, as in the *Progressive Relaxation* exercise above, giving yourself a simple mental suggestion such as "I am letting go of all tension, unwinding, totally relaxing . . ." "Relax, relax, all tension flows away, relax . . ." or any other words you like.

When you have finished the mental tour of your body, remain still for a few minutes and enjoy the feeling of complete relaxation, complete peace.

Then when you are ready, take a deep breath, stretch gently, and open your eyes.

The following exercise using suggestion is based on Autogenic Therapy, a method of relaxation and healing developed in the 1920s by the psychiatrist Dr. J. H. Schultz. It is adapted from Dr. Emmett Miller's audio cassette, "Letting Go of Stress."[6]

In this exercise you make "mental contact" with various parts of your body and give yourself relaxing suggestions as you continue to breathe rhythmically.

Get into a comfortable position.

Close your eyes.

Take a few deep breaths in through the nose, exhaling through slightly parted lips.

Observe your breathing for a minute or two.

Now, let your breathing become a little deeper, a little slower, without straining in any way.

Continue to breathe in this slow, relaxing way throughout this exercise.

With each breath in and each breath out, mentally repeat the following: My right arm is heavy and warm.

After a half minute or so, direct your attention to your left arm.

Now, with each breath in and each breath out, say (mentally): My left arm is heavy and warm.

Now, with each breath in and each breath out, say: My right leg is heavy and warm.

Now, with each breath in and each breath out, say: My left leg is heavy and warm.

Now say: My uterus and pelvic organs are warm, comfortable, and relaxed.

Observe your breathing, calm and regular.

With the next breath out say: "It breathes me . . . it breathes me."

Now say: The muscles of my back and neck are warm and relaxed.

After a half minute or so, with the next breath out say: My jaw muscles are loose and relaxed.

Now, with the next breath out say: My forehead is cool.

Now, with the next breath out say: My eyelids are heavy and relaxed.

Enjoy the sensation of complete relaxation for a minute or so.

Tell yourself: Because I can relax, I can labor and give birth better.

When you are ready, take a deep breath, stretch gently, and open your eyes.

Using the Breath

Focusing one's awareness on breathing is an age-old method of relaxing. It is simple and effective. When you are nervous and tense, your breathing is probably quick and shallow. One way of using the breath to relax is by taking longer and deeper breaths and thinking of tension flowing away with the out-breath.

Get into a comfortable position.

Close your eyes.

Be aware of your breathing. Let it become a little slower, a little deeper. When you inhale, your belly should rise. When you exhale, it should fall.

Become aware that as you inhale you are taking in the life force. As you exhale, tension begins to flow away.

Continue to breathe deeply and rhythmically. Let yourself

become more and more relaxed. Feel your eyelids getting heavier. Feel the space between your eyebrows widening. Let your lips part slightly.

Now imagine that the breath is sweeping over your body like a gentle wave, from the top of your head to your toes. Feel your tension draining away.

As your breath continues to sweep over you, tell yourself: I am going into a more relaxed state of body and mind, deeper and deeper, more relaxed.

Experience the sensation of feeling completely relaxed for a couple of minutes. When you are ready, take a deep breath, stretch gently, and open your eyes.

Circulating the Life Breath

Many practitioners of yoga believe that one breathes life energy called *prana* into the whole body, not just air into the lungs. Directing this life energy to fill a particular area of the body with the in-breath and imagining tension draining out of that area with the out-breath is a powerful means of feeling revitalized and relaxed.

Get into a comfortable position and close your eyes.

Let your breathing become a little deeper and a little slower without straining in any way.

Now as you inhale, imagine that your breath is a golden light filling your body.

Exhale.

Inhale and imagine that the golden energy of your breath is filling your left arm and hand.

Exhale, feeling the tension draining away through your fingertips.

Inhale and imagine that your breath is filling your right arm and hand.

Exhale, feeling the tension draining away through your fingertips.

Inhale and imagine that your breath is filling your left leg and foot.

Exhale, feeling the tension draining away through the sole of your foot.

Inhale and imagine that your breath is filling your right leg and foot.

Exhale, feeling the tension draining away through the sole of your foot.

Inhale, imagining that your breath is filling your pelvic region, the buttocks, and the birth canal.

Exhale, as if you were breathing out through the birth canal, feeling all the tension flowing away.

Inhale, imagining your breath filling your abdominal region.

Exhale, feeling the abdominal area relax.

Inhale, imagining the breath flowing down the spine, filling the chest and back with energy.

Exhale, feeling your chest and back relax.

Inhale and imagine your breath filling your head and neck with life-giving energy.

Exhale, feeling all tension draining away from your head and neck.

Now imagine that your breath is sweeping over you like a gentle wave of golden light. Imagine that it flows from the top of your head to the soles of your feet.

As your breath continues to sweep over you, let yourself go into a more relaxed state.

Enjoy the feeling of being relaxed for a few minutes. Then when you are ready, take a deep breath, gently stretch, and open your eyes.

Using Imagery

Using imagery is a pleasant way to bring about complete mind/body relaxation. This method is similar to the mental imagery exercises in the chapters ahead.

Get into a comfortable position.

Allow your breathing to become a little deeper and a little slower without straining in any way.

Then use one of the following images:

1. Imagine yourself lying on the warm sand at the beach. Listen to the sound of the waves. Feel the sea breeze. Feel the warm sun pouring down on your body. As you do this, let all your tension flow away. Allow yourself to become even more peaceful, more relaxed.

2. Imagine yourself lying on a cool carpet of moss near a waterfall. Hear the sound of the fall pouring into a deep, clear pool. Feel the forest breeze on your face. Imagine that you are giving your tension to the waterfall, letting yourself become more relaxed, more peaceful.

You can also picture tension melting in other ways. Imagine, for example, a little patch of snow melting under the rays of the sun.

In the next chapter you will learn an imagery exercise called The Special Place in which you imagine yourself in a place associated with peace, security, and comfort.

Using Mantra

This is a simple version of the famous Eastern meditation technique of using mantra—the repetitive incantation of a sound or sounds. Many people find it very effective.

Get into a comfortable position.

Allow your breathing to become a little deeper and a little slower without straining in any way.

Then repeat the same word over and over, either silently or softly as you *exhale*. A long-drawn-out OM (*"Oohhmmm"*) is traditionally used. You might want to try the word "baby." Dr. Herbert Benson, author of *The Relaxation Response*, who prescribes using this technique for reducing blood pressure, suggests repeating the word "one."[7] As you repeat your chosen word, let yourself drift into a deeper, more relaxed state.

Checking for Relaxation

In labor it is easy to become tense without even realizing it. But your partner can learn to recognize signs of tension and help you relax. You'll be surprised how much he can help simply by spotting tension and encouraging you to release it.

He can check at the end of a relaxation exercise while your eyes are still closed.

Here are some instructions for him:

First look at your partner carefully. Does she appear relaxed?

Is her breathing slow and rhythmic, or does it seem forced?

Is her face frowning, or at ease?

Do her arms and hands look limp? Are her fingers relaxed, or curled into a fist?

Do her legs look relaxed or tense? Are her toes curled, or at ease?

Lift her arm gently off the floor with both hands, one hand supporting the wrist and the other the elbow. Be sure she is not holding her arm up for you. Her arm should feel limp and heavy as if it would fall to the floor if you let it go. The fingers should hang limply. Lower the arm gently to the floor. *Don't let it drop* or your partner will find it much harder to relax in the future and will be anticipating surprises.

Check the other arm the same way.

Check her legs. Place your hand gently on her thigh and roll her leg back and forth. Do the same for the other leg. They should move freely and feel limp.

Check the muscles in her neck by rotating her head gently from side to side. It should move without resistance.

Don't be annoyed or critical if she isn't completely relaxed. Total body relaxation takes practice and patience.

If you find any tense areas, help your partner relax with massage. For example, place both hands around a tense arm without lifting it from the floor. Massage down from the shoulder to the fingers, asking your partner to let the tension flow down the arm and out as you do so.

Use a similar method with the legs. Tell your partner to let the tension flow downward and out through the toes as you massage.

If her face is tense, massage the area of tension gently with your fingertips.

Use verbal suggestion: "Relax toward my warm hand."

Each time you do one of the relaxation exercises, take the time to turn inward and thank your body for the miracle it is working. Then go ahead with one of the mental imagery exercises in the chapters that follow. The deep state of physical and mental relaxation will give added power and meaning to what you imagine.

∽ CHAPTER FIVE

How to Use Mental Imagery

In the fall of 1984 a young mother made a remarkable discovery that transformed her outlook on birth—she discovered the power of mental imagery to make her labor smooth and peaceful.

Anna was pregnant with her third child. Her first labor had been extremely painful. Though she expected the second to be easier, the labor was so traumatic that she decided she would adopt rather than give birth again.

When to her surprise she found herself pregnant a third time, Anna dreaded the labor. To prepare herself, she registered in childbirth classes taught by Rose Heman, a registered nurse and childbirth educator who had founded New Life Holistic Education Association in Detroit. For six years Rose Heman had been teaching clients how to use mental imagery to cope with labor smoothly and reduce the chance of complications.

During the last three months of her pregnancy Anna regularly practiced imagery exercises like those in the chapters ahead to deepen her relaxation, develop confidence in her body, and create a positive image of birth. After the birth of her eight-pound-six-ounce daughter Julia, Anna said, "I can honestly say I enjoyed labor this time. My third labor was no less intense, nor that much shorter than my second. But I was so able to react to what my body was doing that I really enjoyed the challenge of working

successfully with labor. Mental imagery was marvelously effective!"

Think of this chapter as the beams that support a house. The
beams are its foundation. Likewise, the guidelines this chapter
offers provide the basic building blocks for using mental imagery
successfully during your pregnancy and labor.

Once you have practiced one or more of the relaxation exercises in chapter four, you are ready to begin practicing mental
imagery.

Here you will learn how to create your own inner special place,
a place of peace and security where you can retreat to deepen
your relaxation and feel at peace when labor gets rough. Once
you have learned to do this imagery exercise, you can then
practice the other imagery exercises ahead.

How Mental Imagery Helps You Prepare for a Safe, Happy Birth

With mental imagery you speak to the deeper mind in the
language of images and symbols. Using mental imagery is equivalent to making a clear, positive statement about something you
want to occur. With sufficient repetition you come to believe
the event will happen as imagined. However, the exercises in
the chapters ahead do more than translate positive thoughts into
images. As integral parts of the eight-step method in this book,
they actually help you create the conditions for an optimal birth.

"Mental imagery is a tool of self-direction, not self-deception,"
state Carl and Stephanie Simonton in Getting Well Again, their
breakthrough book in the field of cancer therapy.[1] The purpose
of using mental imagery is not to give yourself an unrealistic or
falsified picture of childbirth. You don't tell yourself that labor
will be easy or that medical care is unnecessary. Rather you
develop a realistic, positive outlook toward birth. You make

changes in your basic attitudes if necessary, rid yourself of self-limiting concepts, and rethink your goals and choices.

Practiced regularly, mental imagery orients you physically, mentally, emotionally, and spiritually to what you have imagined.

Here are some of the ways it works: (Some of the following were already mentioned in chapter one but bear repeating here.)

1. Mental imagery aids relaxation of mind and body so that fear, tension, and the "fight or flight" response don't interfere with the normal labor process.

2. Mental imagery helps you develop greater confidence in your body and your ability to accomplish the reproductive miracle in the most efficient possible way. When you respond to labor confidently and calmly, labor often takes less time, as well as being less painful.

3. Mental imagery helps you surrender to labor so that you cooperate with, rather than resist, the power that will bring your child into the world.

4. Mental imagery motivates self-exploration and self-discovery. As you use the simple exercises in this book, you will probably begin to examine your beliefs and attitudes about birth. You may recognize and release emotional blocks that could otherwise impair a normal labor.

   Reflection is a common by-product of the regular use of mental imagery. A process of growth, it may lead to flashes of insight about subjects that concern you and your baby. You may think, for example, of certain aspects of your diet, your birth plans, your baby's care after birth, and so forth.

5. Mental imagery will create or strengthen a positive image of childbirth, the cornerstone of a safe, happy birth experience. In the fields of health, sales, sports, and many others, we understand that a positive image of the goal is apt to yield positive results. The same is true of childbirth. As discussed in chapter three, a positive image of birth is

a far more important determining factor than knowledge in the overall childbearing experience.

6. Mental imagery inspires positive action. As your mind develops a clear picture of your ideal of a safe, natural birth, you will begin to think of ways to achieve that goal almost automatically.

7. Mental imagery makes you more attuned to the part of you that already knows how to give birth naturally. As discussed earlier, labor is a right-hemisphere process (the hemisphere also associated with intuition, emotion, and lovemaking). Using mental imagery activates this hemisphere, actually helping you bring about a happier, safer childbearing experience.

8. Finally, mental imagery gives you greater faith in your own strength and power and in the labor process.

Basic Guidelines for Using Mental Imagery

Anyone can learn to harness the power of mental imagery to enjoy a more fulfilling pregnancy and prepare for a safe, happy birth. All it takes is the commitment to regularly spend a few minutes practicing.

Before reading further, try these two preliminary mental imagery exercises:

- Close your eyes. Picture yourself holding an orange. Feel the skin with your fingertips. Bring the orange close to your face and smell the fragrance. Then imagine yourself peeling the orange, taking your time, appreciating its texture and its fragrance. Finally, imagine yourself eating a section, letting the juice roll down your throat.

- With your eyes closed, imagine a room in your home. Make a mental tour of that room, taking in as many details as you can, exploring it with a sense of discovery. Then imagine yourself leaving that room and going into another, exploring the second room in your mind's eye.

The imagery exercises in this book are not very different from these except that you will be imagining things directly related to your birth. If using imagery doesn't come naturally at first, you can return to these two exercises and practice them until you get a feel for it.

Read through the following basic guidelines, then try the imagery exercise *The Special Place* on pages 70–71. These guidelines also apply to all the other imagery exercises in this book. Return to them as needed.

- Practice imagery regularly, a few minutes a day, three or more days a week. Be sure to set aside a time when you will not be disturbed, and put all your responsibilities out of your mind for the duration of the exercise.
- Relax. Imagery is most effective when the mind and body are completely relaxed. Do one of the exercises in chapter four as a prelude to practicing mental imagery. Each relaxation exercise in the preceding chapter ends with instructions to stretch gently and open your eyes. Omit this step and go right into whatever imagery exercise you are working with. You will no doubt find that using mental imagery brings about an even deeper, more peaceful state of mind/ body relaxation. After you have been practicing *The Special Place* for a couple of weeks, you may no longer need to do a preliminary relaxation exercise. Let your body be your guide. If you feel like continuing with the relaxation exercises before practicing imagery, do so. Otherwise, just use *The Special Place* to help you relax.

    You can practice imagery in any comfortable position— sitting cross-legged on the floor, in a chair, or lying down— as long as you are relaxed. Wear loose, comfortable clothing. Remove your shoes. If you wear glasses, take them off. Keep your eyes closed throughout the exercise.

You can also try combining mental imagery with rhythmical exercise. Some people find "jogging meditation" effective. In this case a soft, unfocused gaze should replace closed eyes.

- Do the mental imagery exercises with your partner as often as possible. Sit cross-legged facing each other. Or try the "spoon position," in which you lie snugly together like two spoons: Both lie on your side, your partner facing your back with his hand on your belly over the baby. Use pillows under your head and shoulders, between the knees, and wherever comfortable.

  By doing imagery together, you will become more aware of each other's expectations, goals, and plans. In addition, your partner will be better prepared to help you in labor.

  Though it is the mother who gives birth, the father should do the imagery exercises to build his confidence and better cope with labor himself. The way he feels about birth will influence both partners' experience.

- Read the exercise through before doing the imagery. If you prefer, your partner or friend can read the exercise to you while you follow the instructions. The person reading aloud should read slowly in a soft voice, giving you plenty of time to complete each step before going to the next. Another possibility is to make a tape of the exercise and play it back when you do imagery.

  Several guided-imagery tapes are available for use during pregnancy and even labor. One of the best is "Great Expectations" by Emmett Miller, M.D. In this tape Dr. Miller's soothing voice is accompanied by bird song, ocean waves, and beautiful music.

- As you practice the imagery, allow your mind to fill in as many details—sights, sounds, feelings, impressions—as you want. Try to involve all your senses when possible: touch, smell, sight, hearing. But don't be concerned if you don't "see" clear, distinct pictures. Some people visualize vividly in pictures, while others are simply aware of or "feel" an image.

- If you are interrupted, simply return to the point where you left off. If your mind wanders, don't fight it. Acknowledge thoughts as they pass; don't try to drive them away. Imagine irrelevant thoughts as little clouds being carried away by the breeze.

  If negative emotions or images you don't like should arise, simply acknowledge them and go on with the exercise. If the feelings continue, let them come to the surface and explore them. Welcome this as an opportunity to get to know your feelings and perhaps release emotional blocks.

- Feel free to alter any of the exercises in this book to suit your own taste. Change the wording, change the images themselves if you wish. Not everyone responds equally well to the same images.

  For example, in childbirth class the couples were asked to imagine themselves lying on a beach feeling the warm sun. One woman found this image positively annoying. "It makes me think of sweating and sandflies," she said.

  The important thing is that the images you choose are positive and make you feel comfortable. (See the section "Designing Your Own Imagery" on pages 75–76.)

- Give yourself a positive suggestion (such as "I am becoming more and more relaxed") with each mental imagery exercise before opening your eyes. A list of positive suggestions and instructions on how to use them follows on pages 71–73.

- Keep an open mind. Your expectations, goals, and plans for birth may change. This probably indicates that you are learning more, growing, and becoming more attuned to your intuitive mind.

- At the end of each imagery, count slowly to five before stretching and opening your eyes. This is a way to make the transition between the imagery and your everyday life. As you count, tell yourself, "I am returning to my everyday life refreshed, revitalized, and relaxed," or something similar.

The Special Place

In this imagery exercise you create your own personal inner sanctuary, a place of retreat, peace, comfort, and security.

The Special Place sets the stage for many of the other imagery exercises in chapters ahead. After practicing it a few times, you will be able to imagine yourself in this peaceful place whenever you want.

With two or three weeks of regular practice, you will automatically associate your private sanctuary with deep relaxation and a sense of peace. You can then use *The Special Place* as a way to relax body and mind—now, during pregnancy, and later, during labor. In addition to bringing about a deep state of mind/body relaxation, recalling *The Special Place* during labor will help you draw on inner reserves of strength.

Repeat *The Special Place* as often as you want.

Get into a comfortable position and relax.

Breathe deeply and rhythmically.

Imagine each breath you take in as bringing health-giving life energy and each breath you let out as carrying tension away.

Continue breathing this way for a minute or so and feel yourself entering a more peaceful, relaxed state of mind and body.

Now imagine that you are in a special place that is peaceful and makes you feel secure and comfortable. It can be any place at all, real or imaginary: a favorite room; a beautiful natural setting, in a meadow, near a bubbling brook, or by the ocean—anywhere you feel completely safe and comfortable.

Let the details of this special place unfold.

Acknowledge that this is your own place. No one can enter without your invitation.

Take a few minutes to explore this place and enjoy it.

You can return here at any time and feel peaceful and completely relaxed.

Take a deep breath and when you are ready, count slowly to five and open your eyes.

Be creative and enjoy this imagery. Use as many details as you want—sights, sounds, movement, temperature, smell, impressions—using all your senses to maximize the imagery. Experiment and create the special place that best suits you. Many find images that convey warmth especially relaxing—lying on the sand at the beach, feeling the sun while listening to the sound of waves; reclining by a fireplace in a cozy room, smelling the wood-fire aroma and hearing the crackling fire. Or you may prefer to imagine yourself on a bed of moss by a bubbling brook, or sitting by a waterfall, or in an open field, and so on. The important thing is that the special place you choose feels right for you.

If you are practicing imagery with your partner, you can imagine yourselves together in the *special place.* In any case, once you have chosen and created the details of a specific *special place,* share these details with your partner. During labor, when you are feeling uncomfortable and less in control than you are now, your partner (or a friend) will be able to lead you through a guided imagery by recalling the details of your *special place* to help you relax.

Using Positive Suggestions

Wherever appropriate, the imagery exercises in this book include positive suggestions. These "affirmations" are a very important part of the imagery process. They tell your deeper mind what you want and affirm the reality of what you are imagining.

Although using affirmations is quite simple, it is one of the most effective tools for shaping your birth.

Affirmations are most powerful when you are deeply relaxed, because at this time the subconscious is particularly open to suggestion.

You can, of course, use positive suggestions at other times. Some people write one or more affirmations on index cards to be posted in a prominent place. Jeannine, a woman expecting her first child, put a card above her bathroom sink so she could repeat the affirmation every morning while looking in the mirror. Katha, another expectant mother, chanted her affirmations to herself while jogging. Repeating positive suggestions—provided it is done with feeling—can help you replace old beliefs with new and strengthen the imagery process.

Use the affirmations as they are worded with the imagery exercises or pick some or all of those on pages 73–74. If you wish, make up your own. Be sure you are comfortable with the suggestions you use.

In her book *Creative Visualization*, Shakti Gawain writes: "Always choose affirmations that feel totally right for you. What works for one person may not work at all for another. An affirmation should feel positive, expansive, freeing, and/or supportive. If it doesn't, find another one, or try changing the words until it feels right."[2]

Keep in mind that although they are important, there is no magic in the words themselves. The state of mind in which you practice imagery and give yourself positive suggestions and the energy you put behind them are what count.

- Use the present tense. For example, say "I am able to give birth naturally" rather than "I will learn to give birth naturally." This gives your subconscious mind the goal as if it already were an accomplished reality. In effect, all you have to do is wait for it to happen.
- Keep the wording simple. The deeper mind best absorbs

simple, even repetitive, statements. Don't worry if they sound foolish to you, as long as they have meaning and are believable.

- Word all suggestions positively. Use statements like "I am able to labor smoothly," not "I won't have a difficult labor." If you are using a positive suggestion to avoid a cesarean birth, say something like "I am able to birth safely and naturally" rather than "I won't have a cesarean."

If you are unable to believe fully in a positive statement such as, "I trust my body to labor smoothly and efficiently," you can say, "I am *learning* to trust my body . . ."

Affirmations shouldn't act as Band-Aids covering up negative feelings or a negative image of birth. Don't overlook exploring your feelings and developing a positive image of birth (chapter three). "Unrecognized negative visualizations counteract the effects of a positive visualization that people consciously hold in their mind," state Mike and Nancy Samuels in *Seeing With the Mind's Eye,* a book about visualization. "For that reason, it is important to deal with negative visualizations as well as to program positive ones."[3]

Ideally your partner should use positive suggestions with you. This will give him increased confidence in both the reproductive miracle and in his own ability to support you through labor. By learning to use positive suggestions himself, he will be able to help you with them during labor.

AFFIRMATIONS

About Pregnancy
   My changing body is radiantly beautiful.
   I am able and willing to give my unborn child everything he or she needs to grow and be perfect.

I eat nourishing foods for my unborn baby.

I am able to make the best possible choices for a healthy, joyful birth.

About Labor and Birth

Childbirth is a normal, healthy event.

My body is my friend.

I trust my body to labor smoothly and efficiently.

I am able to birth in harmony with nature, in the best possible way for myself and my baby.

My baby and I are working harmoniously together. We are grateful for this powerful experience. *

The strength of my contractions is an expression of my feminine power. †

I fully feel the force of my new life within me. †

I allow myself to celebrate the birth of my child with every sensation I feel. †

I am giving our baby the very best start in life.

The power of birth strengthens me, my child, and my partner.

For the Father

I am able to make the best possible choices for a healthy, joyful birth.

I see my partner as a strong and capable woman.

I am able to support my partner during pregnancy and birth.

We are working harmoniously together. We are grateful for this powerful experience.

The power of birth strengthens me, my child, and my partner.

---

*From the cassette tape "Relaxation and Visualization in Preparation for Childbirth" by June Whitson, CNM.

†From "Great Expectations," a taped imagery by Emmett Miller, M.D.

Designing Your Own Imagery

You may want to create your own imagery to meet your individual needs and goals. If so, keep the following points in mind:

- First read through the eight-step method this book outlines and try several of the mental imagery exercises.
- Clearly define the goal you want to achieve. For success, you must truly desire the goal, believe it is possible, and be willing to picture it as accomplished. However, the goal cannot be fantastic and out of the sphere of possibility (like giving birth to triplets when you know there is only one baby in the womb).
- Be sure the imagery you use makes you feel relaxed, comfortable, and confident. Let your intuition be your guide and feel free to try different images until you find those you like best. Images conveying facts or ideas about pregnancy and birth do not have to be accurate representations of physical objects or events. In fact, metaphors can be quite effective. For example, in one of the exercises in chapter nine, an opening flower represents the dilating cervix. The flower is a powerful and well-known image of the birth passage and, for most women, far more easily imagined than the cervix itself.
- Choose images that *make sense to you*. Don't worry about how closely an image resembles the object or event it represents. If it has meaning for you, your subconscious mind will make the connection.
- End your imagery exercise with a feeling of gratitude and inner fulfillment. This reinforces your goal as an accomplished fact rather than a mere wish.
- Repeat the imagery exercise often.
- Be willing to follow your imagery exercise with concrete action. For example, suppose you are using mental imagery

during your pregnancy to help you avoid using pain medication in labor. You may choose to imagine yourself in a supportive environment coping with labor confidently and calmly, and perhaps feeling gratitude toward your partner for his help in giving effective labor support (the most powerful substitute for drugs). Following up this simple exercise with concrete action might include questioning your physician or midwife about his or her policies regarding medication and finding out whether the staff at your chosen hospital supports natural childbirth, so that you can evaluate your choice of caregiver and birthing place in light of your goals.

CHAPTER SIX

Using Mental Imagery during Pregnancy:
THE FOURTH STEP

As one childbirth educator puts it, you can "program yourself for the optimal birth" with mental imagery.

In conjunction with sound prenatal care, good nutrition, and regular exercise, the imagery exercises in this chapter will help you enjoy a more fulfilling pregnancy, attune to your unborn child, better plan your birth, and inspire confidence in your ability to labor naturally.

The Pregnant Body Beautiful

Everyone's attention turns to the pregnant woman. The glances of people passing on the street linger on her. Friends and relatives are aware of her "condition," make comments, and offer help. Her awesome ability to create and nurture new life seems to radiate a magnetic power, drawing attention from all sources. "Even strangers smile, help the pregnant woman on and off buses, and offer to carry her bags," writes Claudia Panuthos in *Transformation through Birth*. "They open doors, begin conversations, and express congratulations. The spirit is almost pre-Christmas—when the world is celebrating, giving and sharing in honor of birth."[1]

A pregnant woman has her own special beauty, a vitality no

one else shares. Of course, there are negative aspects of pregnancy. Only a philosopher would find virtue in morning nausea. But overall the expectant mother is an image of strength, power, and creativity. She is able to carry twenty to thirty or more extra pounds and still continue her daily activities. And more wonderful, she is able to bring forth a new life.

Look in the mirror and tell yourself your changing body is beautiful.

"I can't do that!" exclaimed one woman. "I'm too fat!"

That's not an uncommon reaction. In our slim-is-beautiful-minded society many expectant mothers fail to appreciate their own special beauty. Obesity is unhealthy. But pregnancy is hardly a form of getting fat! Your baby is not flab!

In many ancient cultures the shape of the expectant mother was held in awe. Goddess figures were fashioned to look like pregnant women. These images in a multitude of forms appear throughout the history of myth and religion. They represent nature—whom we still call Mother Nature—and a woman's miraculous ability to create and nurture new life.[2]

Admiring your body and being aware of the wonderful changes it is working will build greater trust in your body's ability to labor naturally. Take a luxurious relaxing bath. Put on body lotion. Rub coconut oil or some other scented oil over your belly. Perhaps your partner can give you a massage, paying special attention to your shoulders, your legs, your back—any area that feels stressed.

Then put on your most beautiful nightgown and look in the mirror again and remind yourself that your changing body is beautiful.

For the woman who has not already done so, pregnancy is a good time to get acquainted with the sexual organs and appreciate the almost unbelievable changes that take place in the vagina, cervix, and uterus. As a result of increased pelvic blood supply the walls of the vagina shade from pink to violet. Hormones make this incredible organ more stretchable as it gets ready to open flowerlike on the day of birth. The cervix becomes softer, more elastic. While before pregnancy it was as hard as the nose, as labor approaches it feels as soft as your earlobe. The muscular uterus grows to a full five hundred times its prepregnant capacity to provide the perfect home for your developing baby. Intermittent tightenings through pregnancy prepare for the strong, powerful contractions that will both massage and push the baby into the world. With both hands on your abdomen you can explore the powerful uterine walls that now keep your baby snug and comfortable.

The Blossom

In the ancient poetry of India and China the vagina is often referred to as a flower—a peony blossom, a rose, and so forth. An ideal image for both the birth canal and the cervix, the flower combines the qualities of softness, warmth, moisture, and beauty. In chapter nine you will learn how to use this image in labor. Here *The Blossom* (based on a pelvic floor exercise introduced in *Sharing Birth: A Father's Guide to Giving Support During Labor*) combines this lovely metaphor with pelvic floor contractions.

The pelvic floor musculature extends from the pubic bone in front to the coccyx (tailbone) and supports the uterus and its contents like a hammock. This sheet of muscle forms a double ring like a figure eight around the opening of the urethra (urinary duct) and vagina in front and around the anus in back. Exercising the pelvic floor regularly through the last two or three months of pregnancy will increase your awareness of the pelvic region, minimize the chance of tearing during birth, help prevent gynecological problems associated with weak pelvic musculature after birth (such as urinary incontinence and uterine prolapse, an uncommon condition in which the uterus slips down into the birth canal), and improve sexual function and response.

Do this exercise in any comfortable position—standing, sitting, lying, riding the bus, and so forth.

Imagine the birth canal as a flower.

Now picture the flower gradually closing in on itself until it is a tight bud as you tighten the muscles inside the vagina.

When the muscles are quite tight, hold for a few seconds, then, while slowly releasing the muscles, imagine the flower opening petal by petal until it is fully open.

Do this pelvic floor exercise 6 to 12 times or more daily, with or without the imagery, during the last two or three months of pregnancy.

Don't worry if you are unable to tighten the pelvic floor muscles very much at first. With practice the muscles will strengthen. Contracting and releasing the muscles slowly over a period of 10 to 15 seconds or more may also be difficult at first, but you will develop proficiency with practice.

Your partner can occasionally give you feedback about how well you are doing. With a finger inside the vagina he can tell whether or not you are squeezing tightly.

You can also do pelvic floor contractions during lovemaking. Childbirth educators have appropriately referred to this as a "sex-ercise."

The Radiant Light

This imagery is relaxing, vitalizing, and will help you "center" on your changing body, as it makes you feel healthy and beautiful.

Get into a comfortable position and relax.

Allow your breath to become a little deeper, a little slower.

Imagine that you are breathing directly into the womb—where your baby floats in a private sea of crystal-clear water.

After a few minutes imagine that the breath you take in is a soft white light.

As you continue to breathe in, imagine that light filling the womb, surrounding your baby with vitality and health-giving energy.

Continue to breathe the soft glowing light into your womb for a minute or two.

Now imagine that the light which fills the womb is beginning to radiate outward in all directions.

Let it fill your entire body with a radiant glow.

Imagine that the soft glowing light is radiating further and further until your entire body is surrounded by an aura of light.

Keep breathing the light in and breathing out everything you don't need—any tension, any thoughts that get in your way.

Let the aura grow and grow until it fills the room, your entire home if you want.

Breathe deeply and slowly and keep this image in your mind's eye for a minute or two.

When you are ready, count slowly to five, stretch gently, and open your eyes.

Journey to the Center of the Womb

The womb is the center of your pregnancy. It is the heart of all the transformations that take place within you—in your body, your emotions, everything you experience in pregnancy. And it is the source of your labor, your birth.

This brief glimpse inside can inspire confidence in the body and the healthy childbearing process.

Adapt this imagery any way you like to meet your personal needs. For example, if you are preparing for a vaginal birth after a cesarean, put special emphasis on the strength and capability of the uterus.

California midwife June Whitson has found the problems of premature rupture of membranes and waters stained with meconium almost eliminated from among her clients since she has asked them to imagine the membranes strong and intact and the waters crystal-clear. (Meconium is the baby's first stool. Its release in the waters is often a sign of fetal distress.)

Though the baby is growing within the mother, both parents

can imagine themselves in the womb (the father can omit the Radiant Light part of this imagery).

Do *The Radiant Light* imagery (pages 80–81).

Before stretching and opening your eyes, imagine that you are inside the womb and that you have come just to explore.

This is your baby's cradle—warm, snug and secure—where he or she is nourished in your being.

Imagine the baby in his or her own private sea of crystal-clear water, all enclosed by the warm cavern of the strong membranous sac, cushioned and protected.

Fill in as many details as you wish. The baby's eyes are closed peacefully; the fingernails and toenails are growing; every now and then the baby kicks tiny feet against the uterus.

You and your baby are one, right now. Imagine that you are breathing in harmony with your baby.

Let yourself go into a deeper, more relaxed state.

Take a moment to appreciate your baby's home. Notice the beautiful curly bluish-white umbilical cord that connects the baby to the placenta. Through this cord the baby receives everything he or she needs to grow and be perfect.

Acknowledge that as your baby is growing, your body is changing in preparation for birth without your having to do anything about it.

The muscular uterus holds the baby gently and lovingly as it prepares for the powerful contractions that will massage your baby for his (her) first breath and urge him (her) out when your baby is ready.

The cervix is becoming soft and stretchy. It is not ready to open yet. But when the baby is ready, it will open a gateway.

Acknowledge further that your whole being is preparing for parenthood, and let yourself relax more deeply, at peace with the sureness of that knowledge.

Mentally thank your body for the miracle it is now working and will continue to work.

Take a deep breath, slowly count to five, stretch gently, and open your eyes.

The Inner Life of the Pregnant Parent

The day you conceive your life begins to change. Physically, emotionally, and spiritually you revolve around a new axis: your future child. While your body undergoes remarkable transformations in preparation for birth and your baby grows and develops within, you may begin to turn inward.

The expectant mother usually becomes highly sensitive, more vulnerable, and experiences emotional ups and downs. Her fluctuating emotions may be the result of a number of factors: her changing body and hormones; her developing relationship with her unborn child; feelings about impending motherhood; and perhaps because during pregnancy the right hemisphere of the brain, the *heart brain*, becomes more active.

The life-creating months usually inspire self-exploration, growth, and change as both partners confront their future roles and responsibilities. You may find yourself becoming introspective. You may be letting go of aspects of your former self-image. Thoughts about your own birth and relationship with your own mother may surface. Meanwhile your partner may think of his relationship with his father and be concerned about his own impending fatherhood.

The father should be especially considerate, understanding, and accepting of his sensitive partner's highs and lows. But it is important to bear in mind that his life too is undergoing an irreversible change. He too experiences fluctuating emotions. His role is not limited to fulfilling his partner's needs for extra help around the house, for comfort and love. He may need her as much as she needs him.

Some men even share their partner's prenatal symptoms or have symptoms their partner doesn't have—nausea, food cravings, enlarging bellies, weight gain, backache, and so forth. Called couvade symptoms (from *couver,* a French verb meaning *to hatch*), this is yet another dimension of pregnancy that remains a mystery to science.

The transformation to parenthood is bound to be stressful, if not cataclysmic, at times. But the joy of a wanted pregnancy usually far outweighs the stressful parts. Experiencing quickening (a mother's first perception of her baby's movements), hearing the baby's heart, feeling, knowing, celebrating the secret life that is unfolding within more than make up for minor discomforts. The father too can listen to the baby's heartbeat at prenatal appointments. With his hands on his partner's belly he can feel the baby's movements. The first time he does so is often a turning point, when the pregnancy ceases to be a big belly and becomes their child.

A Place in the Heart

Though a person can never know what parenthood is really like until after the baby is born, one can become more aware of one's feelings about it, negative and positive. Imagery can invite potential conflicts to arise so that they can be resolved and negative feelings and fears can be released or minimized. This exercise can help create a smoother transition to parenthood as well as pave the way for a smoother labor.

Get into a comfortable position and relax.
Let your breathing become a little slower, a little deeper.
Feel yourself letting go of unwanted tension as you exhale. As you let the breath out you can also begin to let go of negative feelings and fears you don't need.
Imagine yourself in your *special place*.
Tell yourself that everything that you need to give birth safely is there. (Don't focus on specific things. Just let yourself know all is there.)

Ask yourself: Am I ready for my child to be born?

If you are hesitant in your answer, allow the reasons for your hesitation to drift into your mind. Just let them be there. Don't try to analyze them or do anything about them.

Now rearrange the scene in your mind, making whatever changes are necessary until you see yourself ready for birth and can say: Yes, I am ready for my child to be born.

Now tell yourself: I am an open channel for the birth of my baby when it is time.

When you are ready, take a deep breath, stretch gently, count to five, and open your eyes.

Maternal Intuition

Call it whatever you like—intuition, instinct, inner knowledge, wisdom, the voice within. You are probably closer to your inner resources during the life-creating months of pregnancy than at any other time.

"When a pregnant woman comes in and says something is wrong," states Barbara Pepper of the Midwifery Training Institute in Albuquerque, New Mexico, "I'll pay attention to her even if it isn't apparent to me." Trusting the mother is one of the rules of good midwifery.

Evelyn, a woman expecting her first child, recalls: "While dozing I could feel and see an earth mother figure hovering close to me. She looked very much like the ancient symbols, large pendulous breasts over an enormous bulging belly ready for birth. I realized my instincts were telling me I would soon be giving birth. I accepted the earth mother as my new self image." Shortly after this dream her labor began.

This is by no means uncommon. As Dr. Leni Schwartz writes in *The World of the Unborn:* "During this transitional state, you are integrally connected to the mystery and miracle of the life process. . . . Not only are pregnant women closer to their own unconscious processes, but they appear to be connected to the deepest levels of the collective unconscious. Many identify with the creative power of nature sometimes in the form of mythic Goddess figures."[3]

Unfortunately, as a result of increased dependence on medical professionals and negative beliefs about birth, we often lose touch with our intuitive knowledge. Decisions regarding pregnancy and birth are often guided by convention rather than by a heartfelt sense of what is best. The mental imagery exercises ahead will make you more attuned to your baby and your intuition, thereby helping you better plan your birth.

Getting in Touch with Your Unborn Child

This imagery will help you develop a relationship with your child now, while he or she is still in the womb, so that mother, father, and child are full participants in the planning of the birth.

The womb is the first environment that affects us. Dr. Leni Schwartz, a trailblazer in the field of using mental imagery during pregnancy who has introduced exercises similar to those in this section to hundreds of childbirth professionals through her seminars and workshops, states that such imagery can enhance the family relationship *before* birth. Interestingly, Dr. Schwartz was one of the first childbirth professionals to recognize the importance of the father's involvement throughout the childbearing season rather than just at the birth.

Accepting the baby during pregnancy can facilitate the transition to parenthood. It will encourage you and your partner to confront the issues of impending parenthood early so that postpartum stress can be significantly reduced.

Picture or sense your baby in any way that feels natural while doing this imagery. Don't worry about what your baby looks like in the womb at any particular stage of development or whether or not you are "seeing" him as he really is. Accuracy about anatomical detail is unnecessary. Remember, imagery involves sensations and impressions, not necessarily vivid realistic pictures. It is a language of metaphor.

Do this imagery any time during pregnancy to focus your mind on your baby. The first few times you try it you may find it helpful to do *Journey to the Center of the Womb* (page 81) first.

Relax completely.

This is a special time to be with your baby in a unique way.

Be aware of your breathing. Let it become a little slower, a little deeper. Imagine that you and your baby are breathing in harmony.

Now imagine that you are inside the womb—face to face with your unborn child, who is comfortable and secure in a private sea of crystal-clear water.

Let the love you feel for your child well up within you.

Dwell on the image of your child and on the feeling of love for a minute or two.

At this time you may feel the baby moving, stretching and kicking in his warm, secure home.

If you find your attention wandering, repeat the word "baby" with each breath you let out—"baby . . . baby . . . baby"—and let yourself drift deeper into a more peaceful relaxed state.

Before you end the imagery, tell yourself: I am able to give my child everything he needs to grow and develop.

Then when you are ready, count slowly to five, stretch gently, and open your eyes.

Talking with Your Baby

This powerful imagery can heighten your intuition, making you more aware of your changing body and your baby's needs. It is an excellent aid to making decisions and planning your birth.

Do this imagery any time you wish during pregnancy. (It is not necessary to do it often unless you want to.) You might want to try "Getting in Touch With Your Unborn Child" (pages 86–87) before doing this exercise.

> Get into a comfortable position and relax completely.
>
> Be aware of your breathing. Let it become a little slower, a little deeper. Imagine that you and your baby are breathing in harmony.
>
> Now imagine that you are inside the womb—face to face with your unborn child, who is comfortable and secure in a private sea of crystal-clear water.
>
> When you are face to face with your child, ask your baby what he or she needs most.
>
> Imagine that your baby answers you, not necessarily in words but in images, impressions—by painting a picture in your mind.
>
> Let your baby describe what he or she needs.
>
> Then tell yourself: I am able and willing to give my child everything he or she needs.
>
> When you are ready, count slowly to five, gently stretch, and open your eyes.

You may get no impression in answer to the question that you pose to your baby during this imagery. The imagery can still make you feel closer to your child, sharing emotions that can't be put into words. It doesn't matter whether or not you get an "answer" to your question. The real value of this exercise is in opening your mind to the intuitive part of yourself which knows what is best for your baby.

On the other hand, you may get such responses as a different birthing environment, better nutrition—perhaps even a specific food that should be included in your diet or something that should be eliminated or cut down. Many have a sense of "knowing inside" whether or not the suggestion is valid. You may simply think of love.

This imagery and the one that follows, in which you wait to receive images or answers to a direct question, is called *receptive visualization*. According to Mike Samuels, M. D., and Nancy Samuels in *The Well Baby Book*, "Through receptive visualization a parent may catch a glimpse of the unborn baby and come to know the baby's personality. Even answers to direct questions about the baby may come in the form of visual images or thoughts."[4]

You don't have to believe that you are really communicating with your baby when you do this exercise, although many women do. You may think of the imagery as a means of communicating with your deeper mind—tapping your inner resources.

Exploring Feelings and Needs

Using mental imagery can put you in greater touch with your own feelings and needs throughout the childbearing season and help you make better birth plans.

Get into a comfortable position and relax, body and mind.

Imagine yourself in your *special place* (see pages 70–71).

While in your special place, ask yourself such questions as: What do I really need most right now? Or: What do I most need to do to prepare for a safe, rewarding birth?

If thoughts and feelings come into your mind, let them drift freely. For the moment, just observe rather than react to whatever images arise.

Take a deep breath, count to five, stretch gently, and open your eyes.

If you think of an answer(s) after posing a question to yourself during imagery, try the three following steps:

1. When you finish the imagery, write down the information you received. Examine it in the light of common sense.
2. Ask yourself what practical steps you can take to meet the need.
3. Explore your options, make a choice, and act on it.

Asking yourself questions while in a deep state of relaxation is an effective method of discovering feelings and needs you may not have been consciously aware of. You may think of anything from a more understanding caregiver, more effective labor support, more exercise, to increased closeness with your partner, and so forth.

Don't be concerned if you get no impression at all. This is not a test; there is no right or wrong answer. The imagery is simply a way of heightening one's intuition; it works for some and not for others. The very act of asking yourself the question shows open-mindedness to consider options.

If you feel that something is preventing you from the fulfilling birth experience you desire, you can try asking yourself what is in the way. "What prevents me from having a safe, happy birth?" is a possible question. When you complete the imagery, write down all the answers that come to you. Then examine those that seem to have the greatest meaning.

Sandy, a first-time mother, did this. She had planned on giving birth in a hospital that wouldn't allow her and her husband to invite their friend, though they very much wanted her to share the birth and lend a hand with labor support. At her childbirth educator's suggestion, Sandy asked herself: "Why am I unwilling to make better birth plans?"

Of all the responses she wrote down, one came closest to her feelings: "Because I don't deserve a happy birth." She was unconsciously feeling guilty about an abortion she had had seven years before. However, she was able to bring her feelings to light, acknowledge them, forgive herself, and plan wisely for the birth she truly desired.

Suzanna May Hilbers, teacher-trainer for ASPO/Lamaze, suggests also asking yourself: "What will be my greatest need in the first two weeks following birth?" Preparing now for the period immediately after birth will contribute to a smoother childbearing experience.

Planning Your Birth

Every year thousands of women leave hospitals feeling frustrated, depressed, wishing things had been different. Sadly, many unnecessary cesareans result from poor choice of caregiver and birthing place and inappropriate medical intervention. You can avoid this. The more you take responsibility for planning your birth and the less you leave to chance, the greater will be your likelihood of birthing happily.

To create the optimal conditions for your birth, you must accompany mental imagery exercises with concrete plans. Good labor support, a compatible caregiver, and a comfortable birthing environment are essential to making the method in this book work.

To make truly effective birth plans, you must first have an understanding of labor and a positive attitude toward birth. For this reason the section on planning your birth is here—after these other subjects have been discussed—rather than earlier in the book.

Plan your birth with your partner. Ideally the father should be involved throughout the childbearing drama, not only during its climax in labor. By going through pregnancy jointly, you both will have prepared for a smoother transition to parenthood. In addition, you and your partner will interact more smoothly in labor if you learn about birth and make decisions together.

Be specific about your goals and expectations. Many couples have only vague ideas of what they want. This is to be expected until you learn about labor. But as you gain knowledge, try to make clearly defined plans. For example, if you want to spend time with your baby after birth, don't just say to your caregiver, "It would be nice to spend some time together"; rather, tell her, "We wish to spend at least one hour with the baby immediately after birth without interruptions unless there is a medical emergency."

Outline your goals and expectations as precisely as possible. The less left up in the air, the better.

Be open to changing plans. If you keep an open mind, you may find your goals changing and expanding as you learn more about childbirth. Listen to your intuition. Using mental imagery may serve as a catalyst to bring feelings to the surface, aid conscious decision making, stimulate action, and if needed, inspire positive changes in your plans.

Odd as it may seem, some couples are unwilling to change unwise birth plans even when such may impair their ability to labor normally. Some parents make plans that actually put obstacles in the way of their goal. The best thing to do in such situations is to explore the feelings behind the unwillingness to make plans supportive of a positive birth. Parents sometimes make poor plans for underlying reasons not readily apparent. For example, Renee, an expectant mother in her eighth month, was visiting a physician unsupportive of natural childbirth. "Why don't you change physicians?" asked her instructor. "I trust him," was Renee's first response.

Unsatisfied, the instructor repeated the question and got several more answers: "It's too late," "It will be complicated," until, probing deeper, Renee finally uncovered the truth: "I'm afraid of confronting him."

Renee had always looked upon physicians as authority figures. With the help of mental imagery she was able to see her physician as her hired consultant. Making a simple but important change of caregivers was then easy.

Some couples feel that because of insurance, their location, and so forth, they cannot change plans. However, there are almost always alternatives if one spends the time and energy to search for them.

Leave room for the unforeseen. Prepare for but don't expect complications. If you are giving birth at home, for example, there is a slight chance you may have to be transferred to a hospital if complications arise. Plans for this should be outlined.

Though you may be visiting a caregiver with whom you feel comfortable, there is always the possibility that he or she may not be able to attend your birth. Learn in advance about your caregiver's back-up and make her acquaintance.

"The decisions you make in advance when you are calm, nonstressed, and able to concentrate," states Penny Simkin, childbirth educator and coauthor of *Pregnancy, Childbirth, and the Newborn*, "will help carry you through and guide you and your caregivers at a time when you and your partner need to devote all your mental and physical energies to coping with childbirth."

Outlining your birth plans carefully and thoughtfully is your insurance—your only insurance—for shaping the birth that is best for you and your baby.

Choosing a Childbirth Class

Childbirth classes are by no means a necessary prelude to having a safe, rewarding birth. Good classes can, however, inform as well as inspire confidence.

Speak with a childbirth educator *before* attending clases. Instructors and their approach differ from one another tremendously.

In many cases, what is taught in childbirth classes is the result of a medical view of birth rather than the view that birth is a natural, normal process. Such classes can actually do more harm than good, undermining the parents' confidence and fostering negative beliefs. Likewise, classes that don't tell you how to avoid or resolve possible complications such as cesarean surgery, or that assume all parents in the class will birth within the model of a particular hospital's policies, are often worse than no class at all. For this reason, keep the five essentials of a positive, healthy view of birth in mind when choosing your class (see chapter three). Be sure your instructor supports these ideas.

The best classes are small (ten couples or fewer) and usually take place in a supportive, nonclinical atmosphere, often private homes, where you are free to raise questions and discuss your feelings.

Here are some points to bear in mind when choosing a class: Classes should:

- Meet your individual needs.
- Be held on "neutral ground," not in the same institution where you plan to birth. Though there are certainly many exceptions, hospital classes often reflect the view of the particular institution in which they are taught. Many merely inform expectant parents of policies and aim to create compliant patients rather than give an objective view of available options.
- Present home, childbearing-center, and hospital birth on an equal footing.
- Teach something about cesarean *prevention*, not just about cesarean birth.

Be sure your instructor supports natural childbirth—and not in name only! One way to tell if a childbirth educator supports natural birth is to ask what she recommends to avoid tearing or an episiotomy, what guidelines she offers for children who may be present at birth, and what she teaches about home birth. A true proponent of natural childbirth should cover all these subjects in a positive light.

Imagery to Prepare for Labor

A goal clearly seen is a goal half reached, state experts in the use of mental imagery.

In the following exercises you actually imagine yourself in labor and with your child after birth. Dr. Emmett Miller considers imagining oneself with the child a vital part of the imaging process, as it makes the goal clear to the deeper mind.

Practice these any time during pregnancy but particularly in the final month.

Remember to use the positive affirmations about pregnancy, labor and birth on pages 73–74.

The Snowflake

The Snowflake is something of a "warm-up" to help you appreciate the perfection of birth.

Imagine that you are outdoors watching the snow fall.

Catch a falling snowflake on the sleeve of your jacket. Look at it closely. The snowflake is perfectly symmetrical, an exquisite ice sculpture in miniature. As it melts and disappears on the surface of your jacket, see another replacing it—equally perfect but different from the one before.

Stand quietly for a minute and observe the snow falling. There is nothing you need to do. Nowhere you need to be. But here. Now.

As you watch, the snow falls in its own way, its own time, without your effort. All you have to do is observe the flakes forming endless patterns on the sleeve of your jacket.

Now be aware that the same natural power that creates endless new forms is working right now within your womb, creating a form far more exquisite than the snowflakes: your child.

Tell yourself: When my baby is ready to be born, the door of my womb will open so he or she can be born. It will open without my effort. There is nothing I need to do but let it happen.

When you are ready, slowly count to five, take a deep breath, and open your eyes.

Imagining Your Birth

Imagining the birth and using strong positive statements can help prepare body and mind for birth as well as develop greater confidence.

Get into a comfortable position and relax.

Let your breathing become a little slower, a little deeper.

Before going ahead, tell yourself that this is just an imagery and that your baby will be born only when he or she is ready.

Imagine yourself in your *special place*.

Tell yourself that everything you need to give birth safely is there. (Don't focus on specific things—just let yourself know all is there.)

Imagine that it is now time to open the door which remained sealed so perfectly throughout pregnancy—that it is time to welcome your baby.

Invite those you want to share your birth to be with you: your partner, family members, friends, caregiver, anyone you would like to be there.

Let yourself drift into a deeper, more peaceful state, and imagine that you are surrendering to the power that will birth your child.

See yourself remaining calm and relaxed through contractions.

Tell yourself: My baby and I are working harmoniously together. We are grateful for this powerful experience.

Drift ahead in time. Imagine that your labor is over and you are holding your baby, feeling the joy that follows birth.

Spend a minute or two with your baby.

Tell yourself: My baby and I are grateful for the wonderful experience of birth we have shared.

When you are ready, take a deep breath, count slowly to five, stretch gently, and open your eyes.

Some childbirth professionals believe that using mental imagery not only helps one better prepare for birth, but by linking mind and body may alter the course of labor in ways we do not understand. For example, Kim, a first-time mother, had an unusually small pelvis. Her certified nurse midwife, June Whitson, was concerned because Kim's chances of a cesarean section were high. She suggested that Kim imagine a fulfilling, rewarding birth and tell herself that she and her baby were working harmoniously together and that all would turn out optimally for both.

"Kim went into labor two weeks early," June Whitson recalls. "It was as if the baby knew, 'It's going to be a little hard to negotiate this passage and if I'm going to do it, I better do it now.' The baby was born healthy, at home."

You can also try a receptive visualization to help you prepare for birth.

Get into a comfortable position and relax.

Imagine yourself in your *special place*.

Now imagine the kind of birth you most desire.

For the time being, just let the images come without reacting to them.

Pay attention to those images that feel right and those that make you uncomfortable.

Tell yourself: I am able to birth in harmony with nature, in the best possible way for myself and my baby. (Or use one of the other affirmations on pages 73–74).

When you are ready, slowly count to five, take a deep breath, stretch gently, and open your eyes.

The Ocean

This is a metaphorical way of imagining labor.

Get into a comfortable position and relax completely, body and mind.

Create a scene in your mind's eye of a beautiful natural

beach—a tropical island or anywhere by the ocean that feels just right to you.

Imagine the clear water—deep blue or emerald green. See the waves coming to the sandy shore and receding. Fill in as many details as you want—the sound and shape of the waves, the salt smell, the feeling of warm breezes on your body.

Now imagine that you are out on the water, perfectly safe, floating securely on the water's surface.

Feel the waves rising and fading away.

There is nothing you need to do. Just be here now.

Each time a wave comes, feel it lifting you, gently supporting the weight of your entire body, carrying you along.

If thoughts or fears come into your mind, imagine they are pieces of driftwood being carried away by the waves.

Allow your breathing to become a little deeper, a little more relaxed, as the waves continue to swell and ebb, supporting your body.

Allow yourself to relax on the warm cushion the waves provide.

Feel the waves surging stronger. The waves come, rising, rising, rising, until they reach a crest. Then they fade away.

Imagine that these powerful waves are massaging the baby, preparing him or her for his or her first breath and at the same time preparing you to welcome your child.

Now imagine that the waves are taking you on a journey to an unknown shore—a place where you very much want to be.

Allow yourself to let the waves carry you along, realizing that you and your baby are perfectly safe.

See the shoreline gradually come into view, a place of peace and comfort, a beautiful place.

Allow the waves to bring you gently to shore.

Now take a minute to imagine that you and your baby are together on this shore. Explore your child, letting your thoughts and feelings come as they will.

After you have spent a minute or so with your baby, take a

deep breath, count slowly to five, stretch gently, and open your eyes.

Birthing Together

This imagery for couples will help you develop more effective labor support.

Relax in a comfortable position.

Let your breathing become a little slower, a little deeper.

Imagine that labor has begun and acknowledge that you are together to share birth and to welcome your baby.

Mother, imagine that you are receiving the support you need. If you feel your partner is not supporting you the way you would like, mentally tell him so and rearrange the scene until you are receiving the support you need.

Thank your partner for the support he is giving.

Father, imagine you are helping your partner go through labor smoothly. Tell yourself: I am able to give my partner all the support she needs.

When you are ready, count slowly to five, stretch gently, and open your eyes.

CHAPTER SEVEN

Creating the Optimal Birthing Environment:
THE FIFTH STEP

Giving birth in supportive surroundings is not just a romantic notion. It plays a large part in determining whether or not you and your baby have a happy, safe birth experience.

You create your birthing environment with the place you choose and the caregiver you invite to assist you. (Choosing a caregiver is discussed in the next chapter.) Taking responsibility for these steps is a major, but often overlooked, part of preparing for a happy birth. Choosing carelessly a birthing place or caregiver is one of the prime causes of a disappointing birth experience and an otherwise avoidable cesarean section.

If you have already chosen a birthing place, evaluate this choice in light of the points discussed in this chapter.

The Birthing Place and Labor

You and your baby are influenced by the birthing environment perhaps more than you realize. If you are comfortable and relaxed in your birthing place, you are more likely to labor smoothly and without complications. There will also be less chance of fetal distress and of a traumatic birth for your child.

Animals are instinctively aware of the importance of a secure and comfortable birthing place. In many cases their survival depends on it. For many species, a disturbance can contribute to a longer labor. If the disturbance is great enough—sufficient to make the mother feel she is unsafe or that her baby is not in the best place to be born—labor may cease until the cause of the disturbance is removed.

We can assume that humans, with more highly developed nervous systems, have even more intense responses to disturbances. In fact, as already stated, uterine contractions often slow down, and sometimes stop temporarily, when the mother is admitted to the hospital. This has nothing to do with physical activity—driving to the hospital, walking along corridors, going up and down stairs, for such activity tends to accelerate rather than retard labor. Rather, it is because she is apprehensive in an unfamiliar environment.[1]

Dr. David Stewart comments in his book *The Five Standards for Safe Childbearing*: "How many times have you heard about the lady whose labor began at home with good, regular contractions, who then goes to the hospital where labor stops. In some cases she is sent back home where labor resumes. She then comes back to the hospital where labor stops again. It is a classic story and one told thousands of times over. What is happening?" Dr. Stewart then goes on to cite and discuss twelve different studies that show how entering a hospital induces "maternal anxiety" in the mother which, in turn, causes her body to stop labor.[2]

The same thing has happened in childbearing centers. According to Ruth Watson Lubic, the first year the Childbearing Center in New York opened, many mothers did not progress in labor until they were transferred to a hospital, again presumably because they were anxious in the unfamiliar setting.[3]

Parent-infant interaction and attachment during the period immediately following birth are also influenced by the environment. A mother is extremely receptive to her baby just after it is born. She is also highly sensitive to her surroundings at this time. "Inconsiderate behavior by her attendants, anxiety, and above all separation from her baby . . . may leave an indelible impression," states psychiatric social worker Bianca Gordon.[4]

For these reasons it is essential to choose a birthing place conducive to normal childbearing.

Essential Qualities of a Good Birthing Place

"A healthy woman who delivers spontaneously performs a job that cannot be improved upon. This job can be done in the best way if the woman is self-confident and stays in surroundings where she is the real center (as in her own home)," says Aidan Macfarlane in *The Psychology of Childbirth.*[5]

What kind of setting best supports normal labor? The environment most conducive to the laboring body is that which supports the *inner event of labor.*

As already stated, the laboring woman is especially sensitive. Her deepest, most primitive instincts surface. Keep this in mind when choosing or evaluating your birthing place and you'll be sure to choose the optimal birthing environment.

Following are essential qualities to look for:

Safety. Obviously nothing is more important than your baby's and your health. The best birthing place is where you feel safest and most secure and will receive expert medical care should a problem arise. For some this will be home, for others a childbearing center or hospital.

A setting in which you would feel comfortable making love. "Anything that embarrasses or inhibits the mother's free expression of her sexuality," states Helen Wessel in *Under the Apple Tree,* "adversely affects the progress of labor, for childbearing is a sexual experience."[6]

As mentioned before, labor and lovemaking have many similarities. Both are influenced by disturbances in the environment. A negative emotional climate can make it difficult to birth normally just as it would make it hard to enjoy satisfying lovemaking.

The vulnerable laboring woman knows instinctively, if not consciously, that she is not in an appropriate place for normal birth. Labor fails to progress—the result of an instinctive self-protective mechanism. The mother must *feel normal* for labor and delivery to work normally.

What Sheila Kitzinger, British childbirth educator and author, says of the environment and the second stage of labor applies equally well to the entire childbearing process:

"A facilitating environment for the second stage of labor is similar to the environment which facilitates lovemaking. Although there are doubtless individuals who might enjoy intercourse on the narrow plank of the average delivery table, or in front of a crowd of casual observers, or with a time limit so that if they do not attain orgasm by 4:30 p.m., the act is completed without their participation, or in a stupefying haze of drugs which induce amnesia, confusion and vomiting; those, too, who may actually like intercourse in a windowless, tiled cell surrounded by stainless steel equipment, or under the glare of arc lights, or to receive enthusiastic applause throughout, many people do not appreciate such a setting for lovemaking and may actually find it so inhibiting that it hinders physiological function. We can assume that for most of us privacy, peace and comfort, the opportunity to select whichever position is most convenient and to change position whenever one wishes, the absence of any urgency to complete the act within a specific time, and the knowledge that one shares the experience with someone loved, all contribute to a sense of well-being and to the ease and satisfaction with which the act is performed."[7]

Birth is a time of powerful emotions—fear, joy, and ecstasy. The birthing place should provide a setting where you can express your emotions freely and share intimate verbal and physical communication with your partner. Above all, nothing should interfere with your freedom to react to labor spontaneously and respond to your baby without inhibition.

An appropriate place to begin a family. Birth is immediately followed by a sensitive time for new parents and babies. You and your child should be free to remain together without interruption unless there are unusual medical complications. Your family, including your other children, should be free to be with you and the baby during and/or immediately after birth at your preference.

These are not privileges to be given or denied by a hospital or caregiver. They are basic human rights. However, not all birthing places recognize these rights, and it is up to you to make sure you choose one that does.

Birth is the most significant social event in the lives of most couples—the beginning of a family. You deserve to enjoy this event in an atmosphere suffused with love. Your child, in making the marvelous journey from the cushioned womb to the world outside, deserves the best possible greeting—your waiting arms.

What better way to start a new life?

Peace. The need for peace in labor is undoubtedly the reason, as Dr. Niles Newton observes, that "the time of day when the female is likely to be in a quiet, sheltered environment appears to be the most conducive to labor."[8]

Avoid an environment polluted by loudspeakers summoning physicians, staff chattering in the hallway, instruments clattering, and so forth. This inhibits relaxation and your ability to surrender to the *inner event of labor.*

The birthing place needn't be silent. Some well-meaning birth attendants speak only in whispers which, as one nurse put it, "drives some women crazy." The important thing is that the atmosphere and behavior of those in the environment be tailored to the parents' individual needs. Contrary to the opinion of many books, there is no need to birth "gently" or quietly. In fact, an emphasis on too much quiet can actually alienate the mother from her labor, inhibiting her from expressing herself vocally. Normal sounds such as music, the soothing voice of your partner, and so forth are fine as long as you are comfortable with them.

Your newborn is able to hear inside the uterus and will not be disturbed by familiar sounds, either.

An environment where you are the center of the childbearing drama.
You and your partner should feel that you are in charge, wherever
you give birth. Your wishes and needs, not those of the staff,
come first.

In a good birthing environment you have:

- The right to invite anyone you wish to share your birth.
- Freedom from pressure to use any form of medical intervention that you feel is inappropriate (IV, electronic fetal monitor, and so forth).
- Freedom to do whatever makes you feel comfortable—eat,
  drink, shower, take walks, and so forth.
- The choice of laboring and giving birth in whatever position
  you are most comfortable.
- The opportunity for *immediate* and *prolonged* contact with
  the baby, the opportunity to be with your baby throughout
  the hospital stay, and if there are medical complications
  requiring intensive care, to be present in the intensive care
  unit.

A positive attitude on the part of the staff. "The attitude of the
staff is more important than the physical surroundings," states
Michele Hood, certified nurse-midwife and former director of
Nurse-Midwifery at Booth Maternity Center in Philadelphia.
"A positive attitude is of greater value than a comfortable set-
ting."

We have already discussed the importance of your own image
of birth. It is also important that the staff view birth in a positive
light.

Nurses who believe in the normality of labor and in the mother's competence to birth naturally are far more helpful than those
who look upon labor suspiciously as if it were a medical crisis.
A critical, judgmental approach can unweave even the best-knit
birth plans. Remember that during labor you will be feeling

highly vulnerable. Your faith in your ability to birth normally can be shaken by insensitive remarks.

The attitude of everyone present (this includes anyone you invite) should make you feel confident.

A comfortable setting. Attractively furnished rooms are far more appealing than institutional rooms. But a birthing place need not be beautiful as long as it feels comfortable to you. One of the best hospitals I have visited has simple, unadorned birthing rooms. But the unintrusive health care and genuine concern of the staff more than make up for the lack of homelike decor.

You should have control of the lighting and be able to dim the lights when you wish and, if you like, add your own personal touches by bringing cassette tapes of your favorite music and decorative objects from home such as a picture or poster.

Choosing or Evaluating Your Birthing Place

Whether home, childbearing center, or hospital is the best and safest birthing place is more a matter of personal belief than hard scientific fact. The opinions of childbirth professionals are divided. Some believe all women, healthy or not, should birth in hospitals. Others agree with Dr. Herbert Ratner, former health commissioner of Oak Park, Illinois, who states, "Anything is better than a hospital. Hospitals are for sick people. Being pregnant is not a disease."[9] (See the references at the end of this book for literature about safety in the place of birth.)

The hospital may be the safest place for women with serious medical complications. But I personally feel that home is the best environment for normal birth. Our own first child was born in a hospital. When my wife Jan and I arrived, the only birthing room was in use. Labor-room births, a nurse told us, were against hospital policy. So our birth took place in a dimly lit delivery room.

At the time, when Jan and I were both swept by waves of elation, it didn't matter where we were. But when we left the hospital three hours after our son was born, we couldn't dismiss the thought that leaving our comfortable home in the middle of the night to go to a place for sick people had been an unnecessary excursion.

Our second child was born at home.

"Home is the choice birth place for the normal, healthy mother," states certified nurse-midwife June Whitson, who assists at both birth-center and home births. "Only at home does she really feel in charge of what she is doing. By acknowledging that we feel comfortable helping a woman birth at home, we birth attendants are telling her that we trust her body and trust her instincts to do what is best in order to have her baby in the safest, most comfortable way."

According to Ashley Montagu, "In the supportive familiar surroundings of the home labor is likely to be less difficult and prolonged than it is in the strange and often frightening surroundings of the hospital."[10] Postpartum depression is also less common, largely because an important natural life event is not interrupted by artificial practices and because mother and baby remain together.

The majority of American mothers, however, prefer childbearing centers or hospitals. The important thing is that you give birth where *you* feel best.

Today childbearing centers are widely accepted and offer a sort of halfway point between home and hospital. Most are quite near hospitals on the off chance that a transfer is necessary.

Mushrooming all over the country, childbearing centers offer ideal birthing environments for many mothers. Unlike hospitals, they are specifically designed for birth, are not illness-oriented, and generally embrace a philosophy of noninterventive care. Expert medical care is available, yet the emphasis is on the normality of labor.

To find a childbearing center near your home, write or call the National Association of Childbearing Centers (NACC): RFD 1, Box 1, Perkiomenville, Pennsylvania 18074, 215-234-8068. (Enclose a self-addressed stamped envelope.)

Visit the birthing place and talk to the staff if you plan a childbearing-center or hospital birth. You can't make a sound judgment based on a brochure. Only by visiting will you get a feel for the emotional climate and ascertain whether or not the facility has the essential qualities listed above. Ideally, you should visit several places before making a choice.

In addition, becoming familiar with the environment before your due date will lessen anxiety during labor. The father too should become familiar with the setting so he will be less anxious and able to provide better labor support.

Even if you plan a home birth, you should visit and choose a back-up hospital in the event of transfer.

Don't let your insurance company decide where you will give birth or who will provide care. "Be careful that you don't become confused between 'using your insurance' and 'doing what is best for the baby,' " warns Dr. David Stewart of NAPSAC.[11] It is better to forfeit the benefits of your health insurance than settle for a less than optimal birthing environment.

When my wife and I discovered we were going to have our first baby, we also learned that our health insurance had just expired. This insurance had provided for a group practice attending births at a large hospital near our home. At first Jan and I were disappointed. Later, however, we realized that the lapse of our insurance was the best thing that could have happened. Our birth could never have been the wonderful experience it was if it had occurred with that particular group of physicians or in the hospital where they practiced.

A Place to be Born

The following imagery will help you tap your inner resources in choosing or evaluating your place of birth.

Relax in a comfortable position.

Begin with the imagery *Getting in Touch with Your Unborn Child,* pages 86–87.

When you feel attuned to your baby, tell your baby that you love him or her, you are looking foward to seeing him or her, or anything else that feels natural.

Now imagine that you are able to ask your baby a question and that your baby can answer you—not necessarily in words but in images, impressions, thoughts—by painting a picture in your mind.

Ask your baby: Where would you like to be born? What sort of setting would make you feel most nurtured and welcomed?

Let your baby describe the place for you—the physical space, the sounds, the textures, the temperature, the people present, and so forth.

Let the images take shape in your mind.

When you are ready, take a deep breath, count to five, stretch gently, and open your eyes.

Some people believe they really communicate with their unborn baby. They feel the baby has her own inner wisdom and knows what is needed, giving as an example the way a baby "decides" when it is time to be born and releases hormones from her body into the mother's bloodstream to initiate labor. However, it isn't necessary to believe that you can actually ask your baby a question and that she can actually answer. You can think of this exercise as a way of becoming attuned to your intuitive knowledge.

About Hospitals

Laboring in a hospital is like hiking uphill with a pack on your back. The circumstances often make it more difficult to relax and to surrender to the *inner event of labor*. The very fact that the hospital is associated with illness prevents many expectant parents from viewing birth as a normal, natural event. These factors influence the degree of pain and even the duration of labor.

This doesn't mean you should avoid a hospital if that is where you are most comfortable. You may *need* the backpack. Many mothers are able to labor best and let go only in the hospital setting because this is where they feel safest.

Birth in the hospital can be a rewarding experience. However, it is essential to prepare wisely and take precautions.

Many expectant parents assume that all hospitals are the same or that it doesn't matter where one gives birth as long as proper medical care is available. Nothing could be further from the truth.

Hospital policies and styles of maternity care differ dramatically. In fact, the cesarean rate can vary as much as 25 percent from one institution to another.

We are emerging from an obstetrical dark age. Hospitals are changing. A more humanistic maternity care is evolving. The use of the delivery room is giving way to the birthing room. Fathers are encouraged to attend cesarean as well as normal birth in most hospitals. Many hospitals welcome children, grandparents, and friends to be with the mother during birth. But not all hospitals reflect this progress toward a saner obstetrics.

The powerlessness many couples feel in a hospital with rigid policies often comes as a bitter shock. The way labor is managed in some institutions can rob the mother of her strength and confidence in the childbearing process. Wearing a hospital johnnie, laboring with an IV in the arm and a monitor belt around the abdomen (as some hospitals require) can make her feel like an invalid instead of the radiantly healthy being she is.

You can avoid such disappointment by making wise choices.

The following points will help you better prepare for hospital birth:

- Choose a hospital with comfortable birthing rooms. When you think of it, a hospital delivery room is a rather bizarre place to begin a family. The move to the delivery room is traumatic for the mother (and for the father, for that matter, who often has to change into scrub clothes in a rush). The table is uncomfortable for birth and hardly a convenient place to cuddle a newborn. In addition, if she births on her back with feet in stirrups, the mother's chances of tearing are increased.

  The birthing room (a single room where the mother labors, gives birth, and, in some hospitals, remains until discharge) is far more conducive to normal labor and parent-infant interaction. Giving birth in a hospital birthing room can be a wonderful experience if you follow these simple guidelines:

  Find out the criteria for using the birthing room. In some hospitals only "low risk" mothers are permitted to use birthing rooms. In others, overly strict screening requirements exclude even perfectly normal women, such as mothers who haven't taken hospital classes or those who are planning a vaginal birth after having had a cesarean (VBAC).

  Find out about the rate of transfer. Some hospitals have a high transfer rate—mothers are moved from birthing rooms to labor or delivery rooms for minor or suspected complications as well as genuine medical emergencies.

  Be a shrewd consumer. A good birthing room should offer a pleasant atmosphere, tranquillity, noninterventive care, and immediate and unrestricted contact with the baby. But not all do. "Birthing rooms have become a gimmick for getting people to many hospitals," states CNM Michele Hood. Furnishings alone distinguish the birthing from the labor rooms in some hospitals. And sometimes not even that! In one busy hospital near my home, the birthing rooms are identical to the labor rooms: Both are equally institutional. The care is highly intervention-oriented and loudspeakers blare uninterrupted interruptions to the mother's peace.

Giving birth in the labor room is an option in some hospitals that don't yet have birthing rooms. You may be able to arrange this with your caregiver whether or not it is standard hospital practice.

- Look into hospital policies. These vary widely. Some are rigid. Others are flexible and can be bent or broken to meet individual needs at a physician's or a couple's request.

In some hospitals food and liquids are withheld from all laboring women and IVs are used routinely. In others, couples may bring a picnic lunch and IVs are seen only in medical emergencies. Some hospitals are strict about who is allowed in the birthing room with the mother. Others are not. Some policies just seem to be there—leftovers from a time when maternity care was different. The peculiar policy of withholding liquids from laboring women, for instance, was instituted in an era when many women were given general anesthesia during birth. The unconscious woman might vomit, aspirate the stomach contents, and suffocate. Today general anesthesia is rarely used and in the few cases that it is, the procedure can be accompanied by intubation to prevent such an occurrence.

- Don't be misled by words or expressions like "family-centered maternity care" (FCMC) or "progressive." Hospital birth is a competitive business and many institutions advertise FCMC to attract clients.

Though family-centered maternity care is a valid and important concept, it has become a much abused expression. Some so-called family-centered hospitals actually deny a mother the right to invite a labor support person or the guests of her choice to her own birth. Some prohibit children from the birthing room (as if they were not part of the family!). Some even prohibit children from visiting during the first sensitive hour or so after the baby is born.

A hospital that denies you the guests of your choice hardly views you as the center of the childbearing drama. The excuse that there is no room or that guests would interfere with other patients' privacy is sheer nonsense. Most hospitals that deny a mother the company she wishes have no trouble accommodating medical and nursing students. Don't allow one of the most precious experiences of your family's life to be undermined by such an institution.

- Meet the staff and ask questions. This will give you an idea of the kind of care the hospital provides. Following are questions to keep in mind:

  Are you allowed to labor and birth in the same room?

  Are fathers welcome to remain during all procedures?

  May you invite whomever you choose, including your children, to share your birth?

  Are fathers welcome to attend cesareans?

  What is the cesarean rate?

  Is freedom of movement encouraged throughout labor?

  Are you encouraged to bear down and give birth in whatever position is most comfortable?

  Are you allowed to eat lightly and drink fluids when you wish during labor?

  Are you allowed to bring your own food and beverages?

  Are any of the following procedures routine: enemas? pubic shaving? IVs? electronic fetal monitoring? use of stirrups?

  What, if any, forms must you sign if you opt against any procedure(s) or decide to go home shortly after birth?

  What percentage of women use the birthing room?

  What percentage are transferred out of the birthing room? Why?

  Are you and your partner allowed immediate and unrestricted contact with your baby?

  Are you allowed to room in with your baby twenty-four hours a day?

May your partner remain with you twenty-four hours a day after birth?

- Pay special attention to labor support. Effective labor support is essential wherever you give birth, but particularly so in the hospital setting.

Your partner (or a friend) can buffer the environment by surrounding you with a blanket of love and encouragement. He can also guide you through mental imagery (discussed in chapter nine).

Some couples hire a professional support person (called labor coach, labor assistant, monitrice, or doula) if they are planning a hospital birth. This person can provide reassurance and help coping with labor. If you decide to hire a professional support person, choose someone unaffiliated with the birthing place. This way you can be sure she is there solely to meet your needs.

However, don't depend on a hired labor-support person to substitute for a good birthing environment. Some childbirth educators feel the professional support person should be a consumer advocate, interfacing with the staff and parents. This is undeniably helpful in an institution where having an advocate is needed. But it is far better to choose a birthing environment where such is unnecessary.

The Nursing Staff

If you give birth in a hospital, a nurse or nurses will probably be more actively involved in your care during labor than your caregiver, unless your caregiver is one who remains with a woman throughout labor as do many midwives. A nurse will check the fetal heart rate and your temperature, blood pressure, and pulse. In many hospitals nurses also do vaginal exams to determine cervical dilation. In others a resident or your caregiver will do this.

In some hospitals laboring women and their partners are left to themselves with nurses coming and going as needed. In others the labor and delivery nurses remain with a woman throughout labor, providing one-to-one care. Nurses often provide labor support. "Next to my husband Steve," said Rita, a new mother, "it was the nurses who helped me most. They were so encouraging and suggested things to do when my labor got rough. I don't think labor would have gone nearly as smoothly if it hadn't been for their help."

Many couples prefer a nurse's help throughout. Others prefer to be alone. If you want to be alone, tell the nurse that you and your partner would like as much privacy as medical conditions will permit.

Nurses' attitudes and styles of practice differ from institution to institution (and from individual to individual, of course). Some mothers are pleased, others quite disappointed with the nursing care they received. "It was as if she didn't know the first thing about having a baby," Charlene exclaimed after giving birth in a Boston hospital. "I never imagined a nurse could be so insensitive."

Meet and talk with a few nurses when you visit the hospital. The nurses reflect that institution's philosophy of maternity care—whether birth is approached as a natural event or a clinical procedure.

If you are laboring in a hospital where the nurses don't share your view of childbirth, you can still achieve your goals. But you may have to be more persistent. Be specific and state precisely what you desire. If a nurse insists on a particular procedure that you wish to avoid, be polite but firm about your position. "Dr. Newborn and I have agreed that I will not use an IV," or "My partner and I have researched the subject and don't choose to have an IV."

If necessary, repeat yourself. Don't be intimidated if asked to sign a waiver or consent form. This is required in most institutions when one refuses a routine procedure.

If There Is No Optimal Birthing Place Near Your Home

If they explore all options, most couples are able to find a good birthing place within an hour's drive of their home. But some have to make special arrangements to birth in an environment that has the essential qualities listed in this chapter. For example, Julie and Paul temporarily relocated from their New Jersey home to a relative's home in Philadelphia so they could be near Booth Maternity Center, a hospital known for flexible policies and noninterventive care. When asked later if the wonderful natural birth of her daughter was really worth all the trouble of moving out of state and the loss of income, Julie said, "It would have been worth twice the trouble!"

Perhaps traveling is unfeasible or your choice of birthing place is limited by medical complications. Such special circumstances needn't prevent you from having a rewarding birth. You will simply have to work a little harder to achieve your goals. (For a birthing place or caregiver nearest your home, consult the *Directory of Alternative Birth Services and Consumer Guide* published by NAPSAC. See the Selected Reading List at the end of this book.)

Make sure you have the best possible caregiver affiliated with the particular hospital where you'll be laboring. (Essential qualities of a good caregiver are discussed in the next chapter.) Write down your priorities: no episiotomy unless there is verifiable fetal distress, no IV, remaining with the newborn an hour or so after the birth, and so forth. Be sure your caregiver reads what you've written down and request that it be included in your medical records.

You and your partner might also consider hiring a professional labor-support person. Or, if your partner would rather be the sole source of support, he should be sure to read this book thoroughly, be familiar with the birthing environment, and learn precisely what to do to reduce your fear and pain.

Giving Birth at Home in Your Mind

For most people, the place where they feel most secure, comfortable, and free to be themselves is home. You may not have chosen home for your place of birth. But you can still give birth at home in your mind.

This imagery imagery will help you shut out such things as a clinical setting, medical equipment, an unsupportive staff, even negative attitudes on the part of nurses or your caregiver.

Relax in a comfortable position.

Imagine yourself in your *special place*.

Focus your mind on peace. You can either be aware of the feeling of peace or think of an image that gives you a sense of peace—a lake, a forest, a room in your home, or your *special place*—whatever makes you feel peaceful.

Allow the sense of peace to begin to fill your whole body, your entire being.

Feel the peace radiating from you. Imagine it filling the room.

Now send it to your place of birthing. Imagine it filling the birthing place, surrounding everyone.

Dwell on this image for a few minutes.

When you are ready, slowly count to five, take a deep breath, stretch gently, and open your eyes.

ꙮ CHAPTER EIGHT

Invitation to a Birth:
THE SIXTH STEP

In no other branch of medicine is the relationship between health care provider and client as important as it is in obstetrics. Your physician's or midwife's policies and attitudes can actually spell the difference between whether your birth is a peaceful, natural event or a traumatic clinical procedure.

Read this chapter through whether or not you have selected your caregiver. If you have already chosen a physician or midwife, evaluate your choice in light of the points discussed ahead.

The Caregiver and Labor

A great gulf separates the way caregivers practice. Some, viewing birth as a medical event, actively manage labor by routinely using medical intervention such as intravenous feeding, electronic fetal monitoring, and so on. Others view birth as a natural process and recognize that under all but unusual circumstances the mother will birth normally—and far more happily—without such intervention.

The caregiver will affect not only your labor, including whether or not you have a cesarean section, but even how you feel during the first few weeks after birth. For example, the mother whose caregiver believes in the routine use of episiotomy is likely to be far more uncomfortable after the baby is born than the mother whose caregiver supports natural birth. The mother who spends the first hour or more after birth with her baby without interruption is more likely to have a smoother postpartum period. Some caregivers, however, remove the baby immediately for medical procedures. (This is discussed further in the final chapter.)

Style of obstetrical practice is only one way the caregiver affects labor. As the inner event of labor unfolds, the caregiver can indirectly influence labor's physiology through the mother's emotions. A woman can actually hold her labor back without realizing it if she is uncomfortable with her caregiver (or anyone else in the environment, for that matter). She is more likely to labor efficiently if those in her birthing place make her feel comfortable, secure, and confident.

The caregiver's attitude about the mother's ability to cope with labor frequently affects the mother's own feelings, which in turn affect her labor. Even a seemingly minor negative remark such as "Your labor is going rather slowly" (a common one) can actually upset the sensitive laboring woman enough that her labor slows down even more. If her caregiver treats her like an invalid, she is apt to find it harder to surrender to labor. If, on the other hand, the caregiver respects the mother's ability to perform nature's greatest miracle, this will increase her confidence.

Essential Qualities of a Good Caregiver

The caregiver is a guardian of the natural process, present to make suggestions, to assist when needed, and to intervene only if necessary.

Keep this definition in mind when choosing or evaluating your own caregiver. Selecting a caregiver who sees himself or herself in this light is a long step toward a positive birth experience.

Of course, the main concern in choosing a caregiver—as it is in making all birth plans—is the health of mother and baby.

Should a problem arise you will want to trust your caregiver's expertise. But there is far more to a good caregiver than medical competence.

Here are some other qualities to look for:

A *commitment to natural childbirth* and the belief that medical intervention is something to use *only* if there are problems and *only after* more natural, less invasive methods have been tried.

A *shared philosophy of birth and support of your individual goals.* Labor is no time to argue over whether or not you'll have an IV. The more you and your caregiver see eye to eye, the fewer compromises will have to be made. Having to assert yourself once contractions begin will inhibit you from surrendering to the *inner event of labor.*

The mother who visits a caregiver who is unsupportive of her personal goals defeats her own ends. A woman who wants to avoid an episiotomy, for example, must be sure her caregiver doesn't cut this incision routinely.

Some women prefer a caregiver to take charge and make all important decisions from the beginning of labor until after the baby is born, especially if they've had a complicated pregnancy. In this case, it is all the more important to choose a caregiver who respects your feelings.

A *low cesarean rate.* No expectant parent living in the United States, where one in five mothers gives birth via major abdominal surgery, can ignore this. Although in rare circumstances cesarean surgery can save the life of a mother or baby, most cesareans can be avoided.

The cesarean rate has quadrupled since 1970, from 5.5 percent to an epidemic 20 percent.[1] In some hospitals it is even higher. This increase has a variety of causes for which both health consumers and medical professionals are responsible, ranging from injudicious use of medical intervention to threat of malpractice suits. Thanks to an increasing number of these suits, many physicians will understandably perform a cesarean for comparatively minor reasons in the name of "defensive medicine." That way if there is a less than perfect outcome, the physician is able to prove he "did everything possible."

Many childbirth professionals believe that it isn't so important how a baby is born as long as the baby and mother are healthy. "But there's a lot more to giving birth than getting through the experience alive," as Seattle childbirth educator and author Penny Simkin puts it. Surgical delivery carries greater risks for mother and baby. The cesarean mother has it more difficult all around. After birth she confronts the overwhelming responsibility of new motherhood in addition to recovering from major surgery. She may be separated from her baby, with resultant pain for both. Furthermore, cesarean mothers often suffer feelings of bitter disappointment, guilt, and depression. Many reproach themselves: "Why didn't my body work like a woman's should? What's wrong with me?" Often the problem is not in the mother's body but in her choice of caregiver and place of birthing.

One of the most important ways of reducing your chances of cesarean surgery is choosing a caregiver with a low cesarean rate. What is a low rate? I personally believe there is no justification for a rate greater than 3 to 4 percent. In the 1950s it was thought that a 10 percent rate was quite high.[2] It still is. Yet in the face of a 20 percent average, many proponents of natural birth actually feel a 10 percent rate is, as one physician put it, "reasonably low."

A caregiver with a "reasonably low" rate may be the best you can find in your area. Meanwhile, if you take all the other steps in this book, you will significantly reduce your chance of having surgery.

A comfortable relationship. Your caregiver should talk things over with you in a nonauthoritarian manner, respecting your adult competence and your individual wishes. You should feel free to ask whatever questions you like.

Flexibility. Many caregivers have a "one size fits all" approach to obstetrical care. Someone with flexible policies, however, is better able to support a client's individual goals.

Individual or Group Practice?

Most mothers prefer to be attended at birth by the same person who gives prenatal care. A relationship is developed. One becomes familiar with the caregiver.

If, however, your caregiver is part of a group practice, meet the other members of the practice so you will be familiar with whoever is on call when you are in labor. You might also include a written copy of your birth plans in your medical records.

About Midwives and Physicians

A number of health professionals attend births: Obstetricians, physicians who specialize in delivering babies and the diseases of childbearing women; family practitioners, physicians practicing general medicine and giving health care to the whole family; certified nurse midwives (CNMs), persons educated in both nursing and midwifery who are qualified to provide health care for childbearing women and to assist at normal births; and "practical" midwives (sometimes called lay midwives or simply midwives), persons trained through self-directed study, apprenticeship, and/or through midwifery schools. In addition, naturopaths, chiropractors, and others in the field of holistic health attend home births in some areas.

Note: In some states, peculiar laws prohibit CNMs and/or practical midwives from attending home births. But competent home birth attendants can usually be found despite legislation. However, since "lay" midwives are for the most part unregulated, there is a wide variation in competence and couples should be careful in their choice.

Though midwives are, of course, trained to handle problems should they arise, midwifery is the only health profession concerned primarily with a normal, natural event. Midwives often have a more natural approach than do physicians. This is only a generalization, however. Many obstetricians work with the heart of a midwife and many midwives work with clinical hands.

Many childbirth professionals believe that women make better nurses, midwives, labor-support persons, and primary caregivers than do men. Like the old-fashioned prejudice that kept women from medical school, this is by no means factual. The qualities of a good birth attendant are not limited by gender; nor are negative qualities—there are insensitive caregivers among both sexes.

The sex of the birth attendant is important only if it matters to you.

Choosing a Caregiver

"Rare is the person who strolls into a car dealership, writes a check, and drives the first car in sight off the lot without looking at it," states one childbirth educator. "Yet this is just how many women go about choosing their care provider. They don't interview the physician or midwife to find out how he or she approaches childbirth. Some actually go into an examining room and take off their clothes before they have even met the care provider face to face! It's appalling—the lack of care so many mothers show in choosing the person who is going to help them through one of the most important experiences of their lives."

If this is the way you have chosen your caregiver, you aren't alone. When my wife and I discovered we were going to have our first baby, we began visiting a highly recommended obstetrician. Though she was obviously competent, she used stirrups for every birth and was strongly in favor of routine IVs and fetal monitors. As we developed our own view, we discovered this wasn't the kind of birth we wanted and sought another physician. Looking back on our birth—a peak experience in our lives—we shudder to think how it might have been had we not changed caregivers.

If you are like most expectant parents, you probably began visiting a physician or midwife shortly after you discovered your pregnancy. This is an important part of sound prenatal care.

Meanwhile, as pregnancy progresses, you will learn more about childbirth, think of the kind of birth you want, and formulate definite plans. This is the time to consider whether or not your present caregiver is the best possible one for you.

The following guidelines will help:

Keep the five essentials of a positive image of birth in mind (pages 36–39). We are used to visiting a physician during illness and trusting the doctor to prescribe medications or do whatever will alleviate our problem. Out of habit, expectant parents often relate to a birth attendant in the same way. However, the patient-physician relationship is not an appropriate model for the client-caregiver relationship. Childbirth is not a medical event like an appendectomy in which one's main concern is the physician's competence. In fact, it is the only natural process for which we hire the assistance of a health professional.

If you think of yourself as a client, not a patient, you will have greater confidence expressing yourself with your caregiver and a fresh perspective on the relationship.

As stated before, you are the center of the childbearing drama. It is your birth, your baby. Your caregiver is your invited assistant—not only that, but you pay the caregiver a fee! You certainly have the right to have all your wishes honored.

If the expectant parents remember that birth is a celebration of life, the most significant social event of their lives, they will plan accordingly. As suggested earlier, the parents who plan their birth as carefully as their wedding will avoid much disappointment. It is hard to imagine a couple permitting a cleric to perform their marriage ceremony who said it was against his policy for the couple's invited guests—for instance, their parents—to attend. Most would simply find another person to perform the ceremony. Yet many couples hire a caregiver who restricts their freedom or declares that some of their wishes are against his policies. When you think about it, employing such a person is rather absurd.

Assume responsibility for hiring the right person to assist you in labor. This often inspires self-searching and looking at things in a fresh light.

Most expectant parents who choose a less than ideal caregiver do so because they don't realize how much the caregiver can affect labor. Others sometimes make a poor decision because they aren't mentally ready to give birth for any number of reasons—fear of parenthood, unresolved emotional conflicts, and so forth. It is possible to believe on one level that you want to birth naturally while deep down you are fighting opposing feelings. Taking responsibility for inviting the right caregiver to your birth can bring feelings to the surface and help release possible emotional blocks.

Meet and discuss your birth plans with a caregiver before deciding whether or not that person will attend your birth. Preferably the first meeting should be an interview, not an exam. This applies whether you have just discovered you are pregnant or are in your ninth month and seeking a new caregiver. "The initial prenatal visit is particularly important because it sets the stage for the nature of the care to come," writes Dr. Murray Enkin, professor of obstetrics and gynecology at McMaster University Medical Center, Ontario. "It offers an opportunity for patient and professional to get to know each other as individuals. In addition to the necessary physical assessment, the professional can obtain the information needed to formulate a care plan that meets the woman's needs and desires. In turn, she can make her own assessment of how well the professional will help her meet those needs and desires."[3]

Change caregivers if you are uncomfortable with your physician or midwife. Don't feel hesitant about this. It is always better to change—even the day before labor begins—than to continue to visit a caregiver who does not wholly support your plans.

Don't feel that you must have a completely rational reason for changing caregivers. You may simply *feel* incompatible with that person.

Whatever the reason, transferring is a routine business procedure. Your new caregiver will request the records from the former.

If you change as a result of rigid policies or refusal to accommodate a reasonable request, consider explaining your reasons. Write a letter if you feel uncomfortable speaking face to face. This will make caregivers more aware of expectant parents' individual and very different needs and may inspire needed change in obstetrical practice.

The Invitation

This imagery is an excellent way to tap your inner resources in choosing a caregiver as well as anyone else you plan to invite to your birth.

Get into a comfortable position and relax.

Let your breathing become a little slower, a little deeper.

Imagine yourself in your *special place* or, if you prefer, in the place where you plan to give birth.

Tell yourself that everything you need to give birth safely is there. (Don't focus on specific things—just let yourself know all is there.)

Imagine that it is now time to open the door that remained sealed so perfectly throughout pregnancy—time to welcome your baby.

Invite your partner to be with you.

Then, together with your partner, invite those you want to share your birth to be with you: family members, friends, your caregiver—anyone you would like to be there.

Remember, this is your special place. No one may enter without your permission.

Acknowledge each person's presence individually and thank him for coming.

If there is someone present who makes you uncomfortable, mentally tell that person what she can do to make you more comfortable and rearrange the scene in your mind's eye. If that person still makes you uncomfortable, mentally ask her to leave.

No one may remain without your permission.

See yourself receiving the support you need to let go and surrender to labor completely.

Let the details of this imagery unfold for a minute or two.

Then, mentally thank those whom you have invited for being there, supporting you, and helping you birth perfectly.

Take a deep breath, count to five, stretch gently, and open your eyes.

Sherry and Don, a couple in the last month of pregnancy, did this exercise in childbirth class. When they imagined inviting their caregiver to their birth, they each felt uncomfortable. "All of a sudden I felt I couldn't trust my doctor," Sherry said. "I just didn't want him there. I realized I would never relax and have a normal labor with him present."

Don added, "I think he would have been constantly looking for abnormalities."

They both decided to change physicians the following morning.

Attending Prenatals Together

"A lot of men have a 'well, this is her affair' attitude about birth," states a childbirth educator in New Orleans. "She'll choose the childbirth class; she'll choose the birth attendant; she'll do the reading. And if there's anything I need to know she'll tell me."

Needless to say, the physiological processes of pregnancy and birth take place within the mother's body. She must be examined, not her partner. She's the one who will give birth. But both partners should feel comfortable with the caregiver. After all, that person will be sharing one of the most intimate and dramatic events of their lives. As one father put it, "It's like having a guest share Christmas Eve. You want to be sure it's someone you like!"

Birth is a major life-altering event for both mother and father; the entire childbearing drama, not just its climax, should be shared. "The father should be included at prenatal appointments," states Susan Goldman, CNM. "This way both parents can make a smoother transition to parenthood and avoid big problems during the postpartum period."

There are several advantages to father-attended prenatals:

- The parents are able to interview the caregiver together and decide whether or not he or she is fully supportive of their goals.
- The father is involved at the outset. By the time he sees the caregiver during labor, he feels less an outsider (especially if birth takes place outside the home). He will be less inhibited supporting his partner during labor.
- Attending together, both parents focus on the fact that birth is a major social event of their lives, not a clinical procedure.
- The father's presence often makes the mother less nervous. Many pregnant women feel vulnerable visiting a caregiver. Just by being there, the father can remind his partner that she is not an ill patient but a woman on the threshold of motherhood.
- The father has an opportunity to ask questions and air his own concerns.
- The father is able to feel the baby's position and movements and listen to the baby's heartbeat.

The father will find taking an hour or two from work to be at prenatal appointments well worth it if the caregiver doesn't have evening or weekend hours. He doesn't have to attend every appointment, but he should certainly attend two or three and always meet the caregiver before labor.

Note: There are a few caregivers who don't permit fathers at prenatal exams. Such are hardly supportive of natural birth and can be screened out easily on the telephone by simply asking if fathers are welcome during exams.

What to Do if You Can't Find a Good Caregiver

Perhaps you have searched for a caregiver near your home and can't find anyone who fits your ideals. You can still plan a rewarding birth.

First you can expand the area to which you are willing to travel and be sure you have explored all options. If traveling is unfeasible, there are still a number of things to do:

- Prioritize your desires and stress politely but firmly the items that are most important to you. Be sure to express your needs clearly. One woman in Springfield, Massachusetts, was frustrated because her caregiver didn't respond to her needs when, in fact, she had never stated them.
- Be sure your caregiver has a written copy of your priorities. However, avoid writing a ten-page list. One couple in Boston provided a caregiver with such a lengthy and demanding list, each item beginning with words such as "Under absolutely no circumstances whatsoever," that it merely incited laughter.
- Request to be alone together as much as possible during labor. You might say, "We feel labor is an intimate event and would like to share it in private whenever medical conditions permit."
- Try mental imagery to smooth the relationship. Picture your relationship with your caregiver the way you would like it to be. See yourself face to face with her discussing your needs and wishes effortlessly. Imagine your caregiver listening and responding positively. Mentally thank her for con-

sidering your needs. This exercise works in some situations and has been used in business to smooth rocky relationships between employees and supervisors. If nothing else, it may give you greater confidence in expressing yourself.

Some couples choose to be alone (or only with family) during birth because they feel it is a private event that shouldn't be shared with a professional. Others birth without assistance because they cannot find a caregiver who supports their plans—to birth at home, for example. David and Lee Stewart could not find a physician or midwife to attend any of their five home births (which took place between 1962 and 1976). Accordingly, their five healthy children were all born at unattended births. (However, the Stewarts don't suggest that others follow their example.)

Inspired by the need for parents to have choices in childbirth, David and Lee later founded the National Association for Parents and Professionals for Safe Alternatives in Childbirth (NAPSAC), which now has one hundred chapters in twenty-two countries and ten thousand members. Today NAPSAC publishes nine books, several pamphlets, and a quarterly newsletter, which promote safe, natural birth (see the Selected Reading List at the end of this book).

If you want to birth at home but are unable to find a caregiver, consult the NAPSAC *Directory of Alternative Birth Services and Consumer Guide* (see the Selected Reading List).

About Medical Intervention

"Childbirth in itself is a natural phenomenon," says Dr. G. J. Kloosterman, professor of obstetrics at the University of Amsterdam, "and in the large majority of cases needs no interference whatsoever—only close observation, moral support, and protection against human meddling."

While *appropriate intervention* has saved the lives of mothers and babies and carries benefits that outweigh the risks, *inappropriate intervention* carries risks that outweigh the benefits.

Today many people feel that *routine* intervention is appropriate. A conscientious resident in a New York hospital once told me: "I can't understand why so many couples object. I would never allow my own wife to labor without continuous electronic monitoring." Many parents feel the same. "I felt secure knowing my baby's heart was constantly recorded," said one mother. Her husband thought the machine was great because a graph showed him each time a contraction was beginning. Thanks to such views, the monitor and other interventions, originally designed for complicated labors, have now become routine in many American hospitals.

However, all forms of medical intervention, from fetal monitoring to obstetrical pain medication, can inhibit the labor process.

Injudicious use of medical intervention can trigger a vicious spiral culminating in cesarean surgery. The following example is a common sequence in American hospitals: A mother's labor flags (perhaps because she is anxious as a result of electronic fetal monitoring, an IV, the hospital environment, or all put together). She is given Pitocin, a hormonal solution to augment contractions. The hormonally augmented contractions are more painful and the mother requires medication. This in turn causes her contractions to slow further. More Pitocin is administered until fetal distress is recorded and the mother is operated on. Avoiding all forms of inappropriate intervention is one of the most important steps in cesarean prevention.

Most proponents of natural childbirth agree that medical intervention is appropriate only if there are genuine complications and *only after* less invasive, natural means have been tried first. This is a good rule of thumb to keep in mind (except in rare emergencies). Say, for example, that labor is flagging. One tries all the natural means to get it going: drinking additional fluids, walking, position changes, showers, massage, change of environment, using mental imagery, nipple stimulation, and love-making. If all these fail (not likely), *then* it might be appropriate to consider Pitocin.

Medical intervention also influences the *inner event of labor* and thereby alters labor's physiology in ways that are not always apparent. As already stated, labor is a sexual experience and the same conditions that influence lovemaking affect the physiology of labor. The mother finds it hard to surrender to labor while surrounded by attendants who act as if birth were a disaster waiting to happen, just as she might find it hard to surrender to lovemaking under the same conditions.

Pain Medication

No medication has been proven entirely safe for the baby. It can impair labor and increase the possibility of other interventions such as hormonal augmentation and forceps delivery. As Grantly Dick-Read points out, medicated women also "fail to experience the elation that often follows birth."[4] Depending on the type and amount of the medication, the mother may be less able to relate to her infant after birth.

The need for medication varies depending on the individual labor. As a result of several factors, some labors are more painful than others. Only the laboring woman knows how she feels. Therefore, the decision whether or not to use medication must be hers and hers alone.

A woman often asks for medication toward the end of first stage, when contractions are usually difficult and she is feeling most vulnerable. When a woman asks for medication at this time, often what she needs is reassurance and support. Her partner can reduce the fear and pain of labor tremendously. All natural methods of pain relief should be tried before resorting to medication. Those who had hoped to avoid drugs are frequently disappointed after birth if they took medication at a time when they were feeling vulnerable.

There are four basics in successfully avoiding medication, according to Penny Simkin, author of *Pregnancy, Childbirth, and the Newborn:*

1. Motivation on the part of the mother. She must want to give birth without medication.
2. Emotional support from the partner and the staff.
3. Knowing what to expect and how to cope with labor.
4. An uncomplicated labor.

Should one of these ingredients be missing, the chances for an unmedicated birth are still good—for example, if the woman's motivation is flagging but she has excellent support, or if she is poorly prepared but strongly desires to birth naturally.

If you want to avoid medication in the hospital, tell the nurse your plans and request that she avoid recommending medication. If you change your mind, you can ask for it.

Episiotomy

The episiotomy is an incision made to enlarge the birth outlet as the baby is born. The alleged advantages include: substituting a neat cut for a ragged tear, the cut being easier to suture; shortening second stage; and reducing gynecological problems after birth. No convincing evidence supports the latter claim and certainly nothing justifies the near 100 percent episiotomy rate of many physicians.

Perhaps an episiotomy is indicated in unusual cases when it is advisable to complete the delivery quickly, and some might add when a large tear is threatened. *Small* tears, however, are always preferable to an episiotomy. The idea of substituting a larger, neater cut for a small ragged tear—which in many cases needs no stitching—is absurd.

The stitched episiotomy site is uncomfortable for days, even weeks, after the baby is born, and the mother should make every effort to avoid it.

Minimizing your chance of undergoing an episiotomy is largely a matter of choosing a caregiver who does not do this incision unless there is an emergency.

Your chances of tearing will be greatly reduced by:

- Following the eight steps in this book, particularly choosing a peaceful birthing environment and a good caregiver.
- Avoiding the supine position with legs in stirrups.
- Doing *The Blossom* (pages 79–80) throughout the final trimester.
- Practicing perineal massage.
- Applying warm compresses to the perineum during second stage. Your partner or caregiver can do this.

Other Labor Helpers

Today most fathers remain with their partner throughout labor. The father is able to provide invaluable support as well as share the birth of his child.

Some couples also invite family and friends to their birth. Provided everyone has a positive attitude, this can create a wonderful festive atmosphere. The very presence of a family member or friend can be a form of labor support, even if he or she does nothing but share the event.

An additional person or people can lend a hand as well. For example, a woman's mother or friend can relieve the father; someone else can prepare light meals and beverages. Children can make their own special contributions and can be given small tasks—bringing fresh sheets for the mother, a cool washcloth for her forehead, and so forth.

Birth through a child's eyes can add a unique kind of magic to the miracle. Children, of course, should be prepared in advance for birth so that they will not be surprised by the mother's behavior or by the sight of blood.

If the mother has no partner, or if her partner is unable to attend the birth, she should be sure to have someone with her to give her emotional and physical support during this especially vulnerable time. (Labor support is briefly discussed in the next chapter.) This is so important to the outcome of a natural birth that one physician I know won't accept clients who don't plan to have someone present during labor.

Though hospital nurses sometimes give excellent support, a nurse is no substitute for the mother's own support person. Nursing shifts change and the mother may have several different attendants. Besides, the support person should not be affiliated with the birthing place (to ensure that he or she is present solely to meet the mother's needs), and the mother should know or at least meet with the support person before labor.

A relative, friend, or childbirth educator can provide labor support. Women who have experienced birth often make good support persons because they are able to share their personal feelings. Carol invited a friend who had given birth to two children to help her during her first labor. "During early labor we spent most of the time chatting and looking at pictures of her daughters. I didn't feel I was in any great need of support. But it was reassuring to know that a friend was there. However, when labor got rough, about the time I was six centimeters dilated, I needed her with me every minute. Just hearing her tell me 'I know it's hard, but you can do it' meant the world to me. I don't know how I would have managed alone."

Having given birth, however, is not an essential for helping someone through labor. Ruth's partner was out of state when she went into labor. "I missed his presence at the birth terribly," she said, "but I made other arrangements for support. I invited my friend Gary to be with me. I felt it was important to have a male friend there to add a sense of balance and wholeness and to give me needed strength at a time when I would be dependent.

"It was amazing how much I depended on Gary. When contractions began I felt as if I were holding my labor back psychologically. Then as soon as he arrived, the contractions picked up.

"Gary didn't coach me with 'Breathe one, two, three, push, push' or whatever coaches say. He just sat by my side, holding my hand and keeping up steady eye contact. That's what I really needed. That's what helped me get through labor."

ᘓ CHAPTER NINE

Using Mental Imagery in Labor:
THE SEVENTH STEP

*F*inally labor has begun. A woman and man will become mother and father, greeting the child they have so long anticipated.

For some, the childbearing miracle may creep up softly and those first few contractions seem like bare whispers across the uterus. At first the mother may not even realize she is in labor. "Has the time actually come?" many parents-to-be ask themselves. "Is this really labor?"

Most labors begin slowly and contractions build in intensity as labor progresses. For some, however, labor heralds its onset with the suddenness of a thunderclap. My wife Jan's first labor began with cataclysmic fury. Contractions rolled onward with barely two to three minutes between them. Labor was short, only six hours or so, but intense.

Regardless of how labor begins or how long it lasts, for most parents it is an exciting time. And for all parents it is a life-altering event.

Signs That Labor May Soon Begin

You may experience all, some, or none of these signs prior to labor.

Engagement or *lightening.* For first time mothers, the baby usually drops further into the pelvis (the head is said to *engage*) one to three weeks before birth. This is accompanied by *lightening;*

in other words, less pressure on the ribs and less shortness of breath. For those who have previously had children, engagement may not occur until labor.

Discharge of the mucus plug. The thick glob of mucus that filled the cervix and sealed the uterus is often tinged with blood from the cervical capillaries. This is often an exciting sign—as if the uterus were uncorking for the big event. Discharge of the mucus plug often occurs twenty-four to forty-eight hours before labor, but may occur a week or more before birth, during labor, or may not be noticed at all.

Increase in Braxton-Hicks contractions. These mild contractions, named after the physician who first described them, occur throughout pregnancy but often increase in frequency and intensity just prior to labor's onset.

Prelabor diarrhea often but not always empties the bowels before birth.

Membranes may rupture and water may be discharged in a trickle or a gush. In about 10 to 15 percent of mothers, this occurs before labor's onset (within forty-eight hours). Otherwise, membranes rupture during labor. If membranes rupture before labor begins, notify your caregiver.

Nesting instinct. A day or two before labor begins, the mother

FIRST STAGE:	cervical effacement (thinning) and dilation (opening) average length: 12 hours
SECOND STAGE:	birth average length: 1-2 hours
THIRD STAGE:	delivery of the placenta average length: 10-15 minutes

often feels a sudden urge to clean house and prepare a place for her child.

A *spurt of energy* may also precede labor's onset.

An *intuition that labor is soon to begin* may be felt by either or both parents.

Using Mental Imagery in Labor

"Mental imagery may not take all the pain away from labor," states Loretta Ivory, director of the Denver Birthing Center, "but one thing I've learned in my practice: it reduces that pain quite dramatically!"

Mental imagery will also help you relax and surrender to labor, and in some cases actually make labor contractions more effective. As stated earlier, using mental imagery will make you a partner rather than an adversary of the life-creating force.

"When a person deliberately concentrates on a relaxed, peaceful image, a number of physiological changes take place," write Mike and Nancy Samuels in *The Well Baby Book.* "Muscles relax, heart rate and blood pressure decrease, oxygen consumption of cells decreases, and respiratory rate decreases. Basically an opposite set of physiological changes takes place when a person concentrates on a frightening or stressful image."[1] Mental imagery can keep you from experiencing the fight-or-flight response that can make labor contractions more painful.

As the *inner event of labor* unfolds, it is as if the uterine contractions open a channel to your instinctive mind. This is another reason mental imagery—which influences the instinctive mind—is an ideal tool for coping with labor.

Using imagery in labor will prove most effective if you have practiced the exercises in this book throughout the latter months of pregnancy and, most important, have followed all the other steps. But you can still use imagery effectively even if you are picking up this book during labor.

POSITIONS FOR LABOR

Labor in whatever position you are comfortable and change positions as desired.

However, avoid back-lying. In this position the uterus depresses major arteries, diminishing blood and oxygen supply to the baby.

First Stage

Upright positions—standing, sitting in a rocking chair, and so forth—often make labor less uncomfortable and more efficient.

Walking shortens labor, as gravity helps dilate the cervix. When a contraction occurs, lean against the wall or your partner.

Second Stage

The following are most comfortable and efficient for the majority of mothers. Again, change position as often as you like. If your caregiver is unfamiliar with delivering a baby with the mother squatting, on hands and knees, and so forth, you can always change position just before birth.

- Side-lying with partner supporting one leg or mother drawing both legs toward belly. (A natural sleeping position in which the pelvic musculature is usually more relaxed.)
- Sitting on birthing chair or toilet. (The most comfortable position for many women.)
- Semisitting in bed with back well supported by pillows.
- On hands and knees, resting on elbows and knees, or with head and chest on a pillow between contractions. (Helpful for backache, breech baby, or other difficult delivery.)

- Squatting with partner's support, sitting or reclining between contractions. (Presents largest pelvic diameter to the baby; especially good for long and difficult second stage.)
- Standing, leaning against wall or partner.

Avoid stirrups. Legs in stirrups will make pushing more difficult and increase your chances of tearing and forceps delivery. (Using stirrups became popular when many women were unconscious during birth.)

You'll probably find imagery most effective once labor becomes active. However, you can use the exercises in this chapter any time you wish during both the first and second stages.

Do any or all of the following exercises. Or create your own. If you design your own imagery, be sure it is something that is relaxing and makes you feel comfortable (see page 75). You can do the imagery yourself, or your partner, speaking in a soothing voice, can guide you. For optimal results, it is essential to combine imagery with labor support, discussed further along in this chapter.

The Special Place

Imagine yourself in your *special place* (pages 70–71). This personal sanctuary is associated with peace and relaxation, all the more so if you have practiced this imagery through the last trimester.

Some find the *special place* helpful during first-stage contractions. You may want to do this imagery during some contractions and just be with your partner during others.

Your partner can guide you with the imagery, reminding you of the details. For example, Neil, whose partner's *special place* was a clearing in a forest by a bubbling brook, said: "Imagine yourself lying on the soft moss. You can hear the rushing water playing over the rocks, the songs of the birds in the birch trees around. There is a faint smell of pine in the air. Sense the peace of this place. Let yourself relax, let go. . . ."

The *Special Place* is particularly helpful if there are disturbances in the environment. Jackie was unexpectedly transferred from her home to the hospital as a result of a minor complication. She found this imagery effective in smoothing what might otherwise have been a traumatic transition. "I felt that my baby and I were going to our *special place* where we would be undisturbed."

Another couple got wholly involved in this imagery. Their *special place* focused on a trip they planned to a south sea island after the baby was born. They brought posters of this island into the birthing room, played island music, and used coconut shells for drinking glasses. They even hung a bikini near the bed to remind the mother she would soon regain her prepregnant shape.

The Opening Flower

Many midwives instruct laboring women to visualize the cervix opening with each contraction. Some mothers can do this easily, while others have difficulty. One laboring woman said: "All I can think of is this yucky thing!" In this imagery, instead of thinking of the cervix or birth canal, you think of an opening flower. Your mind will make the connection.

The opening flower is the ideal metaphor for the dilating cervix and birth canal, for it combines the elements of wetness, warmth, unfolding, and beauty. In fact, many have compared the opening vagina to a flower blooming. A universal image used throughout the world, this is one of the most powerful and effective symbols to imagine during both first stage (when the cervix opens) and second stage (when the vagina unfolds).

Imagine a beautiful flower. Choose any flower you want— a rose, a lily, even the thousand-petaled lotus so often figured in Oriental imagery—as long as it is beautiful to you.

Imagine that it is gradually expanding petal by petal until it is fully opened.

You can add as much detail as you want: dew on the petals, warm sun rays, fragrance, and so forth. You can even picture or sense yourself standing in a garden surrounded by hundreds of flowers and imagine that you have chosen this one special opening flower to observe.

For many, the *opening flower* is the most effective imagery. For example, Charlotte was having a long and difficult labor with her first child. A nurse had tried everything to help her: massage, compresses, a bath. She had walked along the corridor with her, hoping that gravity would help dilate the cervix. But Charlotte remained at 8 cm. for some reason. "I can't do it," she said, on the verge of tears.

Earlier in the day the nurse had attended a mental imagery workshop. It was the first time she had ever heard of using imagery in labor. One of the images stood out in her mind: an opening flower. She started talking about this image with the frustrated mother to pass the time. "Let's think of a beautiful garden of roses," she said. "The early morning sun is warming the flowers. Imagine them blooming."

Charlotte did the imagery through the next few contractions. She didn't look as tense. She stopped talking about her frustration and her inability to go through labor.

"Now let's imagine one perfect rose just ready to bloom," the nurse said. "It has little dewdrops on it; it's very soft and very beautiful. Imagine it opening."

Another contraction.

"The petals are opening wider and wider," the nurse continued. "Imagine the rose coming into full bloom."

Suddenly Charlotte started pushing—right there in the corridor. The nurse barely had time to get her back into the labor room before the baby was born.

Her cervix had opened just like the rose. *

Note: You can also do the Opening Flower imagery during pregnancy. In this case, think of the opening flower as a symbol of yourself opening on all levels—mentally, emotionally, and spiritually—to a joyful birth and to parenthood.

The Waterfall

Focus your mind on the image of a waterfall pouring into a stream. Give your tension to the waterfall. See the stream flowing effortlessly over its rocky bed.

You can fill in more details if you wish. You can hear the sound of the fall, feel a fine spray of water on your face, see a grove of trees surrounding the stream, and so on.

Now imagine that your body is like the stream, able to flow along with labor and give birth effortlessly just as the stream flows along as if by its own power.

The Ocean

Labor contractions are often compared to waves. Each rises, reaches a crest, and ebbs away.

Focus your mind on the ocean. Imagine waves rising and ebbing away.

Fill in any details you want—the warm sun, the salt air, the sea breeze, and so forth.

Now think of your contractions like the waves, rising and falling. Tell yourself that you are able to flow along with the waves and float with their movement.

Imagining the Birth

For many mothers, envisioning the physical details of the birth helps labor progress more smoothly and rapidly. Loretta Ivory's

---

*This story is from Suzanna May Hilbers, teacher-trainer for ASPO.

clients at the Denver Birthing Center, for example, find this simple imagery an effective way to cooperate with the sensations of labor.

Imagine yourself opening. Envision the baby's head against the cervix and the cervix widening to let it pass.

At the same time, mentally say yes to the contractions as they come and fade away.

Remind yourself that the more powerful contractions are the most effective. They massage and stimulate the baby as they open the birth passage and push the baby downward.

With each contraction imagine the baby moving through the birth passage, closer and closer to your waiting arms.

Shawne, a mother who used this imagery, said: "The imagery changed automatically during labor. Through most of first stage I was seeing myself opening and focusing on the opening sensations of early labor. With the downward sensations of transition, I visualized my baby going deeper into the pelvis and traveling along the birth canal."

Laboring women find all sorts of images effective. Imagery can be a means of attuning to labor or simply focusing the attention on something else. *The Opening Flower, The Ocean,* and *Imagining the Birth* all reflect the labor process. Some mothers, however, design images that seem to have no connection with labor. Yet for them these images are relaxing and effective means of coping with contractions. Suzanna May Hilbers related the following example:

One couple focused their attention on fruit picking. Sitting on the labor bed next to his wife, the husband painted a vivid verbal picture of picking raspberries and strawberries and occasionally counting the berries as they were put into a pail. Interestingly, the mother found this image relaxing only when her husband picked the fruit. Imagining herself picking took her energy away from labor.

Be creative! Do whatever you like with mental imagery. Any image that works for you is a good image. Explore new worlds.

Labor is hard work. But you can enjoy it.

Using the Breath

Many childbirth educators teach breathing patterns as a way to focus or distract attention during contractions. Breathing techniques vary from simple abdominal breathing to complex patterns. They are tools to use only if you personally find them effective.

Laboring women have varying degrees of success with breathing patterns. Regulated breathing can be effective for some while for others it is merely an added inconvenience. As Kathy, a childbirth educator from St. Paul, Minnesota, said: "Though some mothers find breathing patterns extremely helpful, they didn't help me in the least! I found it far more effective to groan and moan during difficult contractions and just imagine myself opening."

Slow rhythmic breathing can be an effective tool for relaxation in labor just as it aids difficult physical endeavors such as long-distance jogging and hiking. On the other hand, the complex breathing patterns taught in some childbirth classes can actually impair labor by exhausting the mother and preventing her from surrendering to the process.

Unfortunately, in the interest of a more natural approach to labor, some childbirth professionals condemn all forms of breathing as useless. However, the fact of the matter is that breathing patterns help some and do not help others. Any breathing pattern is a good one if it helps you. Some mothers find even the more artificial patterns designed purely for distraction useful—especially if they have used distraction to deal with physical stress all their lives.

This book includes only slow, relaxing breathing because you will probably find additional patterns unnecessary if you follow all the eight steps carefully. Combined with imagery, controlled slow rhythmic breathing helps you attune to labor and draw on inner reserves of strength.

The Cleansing Breath

Often taught in childbirth classes, the cleansing breath is a long deep audible breath (usually in through the nose and out the mouth) done at the beginning and end of each contraction. It tells others that a contraction is beginning or ending. Meanwhile, you can imagine this breath revitalizing your body, cleansing your mind of negative thoughts, and helping you tune in to the labor process.

The Golden Breath

Practice *The Golden Breath* during pregnancy and, if you find it helpful, use it as a means of focusing your attention during labor.

Breathe slowly, deeply, and rhythmically. As you do so, imagine the in breath as a soft golden light, giving you energy and revitalizing you. You can imagine the soft golden light entering your womb or sweeping through your entire body, whichever you prefer.

Imagine the out breath draining away all tension, fear, and negative thoughts.

Sigrid, a mother of two in the San Jose, California, area, found a simple variation of this imagery, without focusing attention on accompanying rhythmic breathing, extremely effective. (She had thought of the imagery spontaneously during her first labor.)

"At first a contraction felt like a tight dark knot," she said. "But when I imagined turning it to gold, the pain started flowing away."

Her husband, Richard, guided her with this imagery. When a contraction began, he would say, "Turn the contraction to gold. See the gold shimmering and glowing."

"I'm beginning to see it. Now it's almost all gold. It's all gold," she said during one contraction.

If she was completely overwhelmed and said, "I can't do that," Richard would tell her to turn a little bit of the contraction to gold. Once she was able to do this, she would imagine a little more of the dark knot turning to gold, and so forth.

You can breathe rhythmically through one contraction and simply relax and be with your partner or use mental imagery through another. The best approach is flexibility. Do whatever feels best at the time.

Some find chanting effective in addition to or as an alternative to rhythmic breathing. Indian healing ceremonies are often conducted with chanting, which brings about a state of reverie. For some the state of reverie facilitates using mental imagery. Actually the monotonous *haa-hoo* (pant/blow) breathing taught in some childbirth classes has an almost chantlike quality. Since the mother tends to breathe rapidly, however, it can be rather exhausting.

If you chant, use any sound that makes you feel relaxed and comfortable—a simple word or mantra, the word *om* or even *baby* on the out-breath.

Bearing Down in Second Stage

The urge to bear down varies with different mothers. It may be quite forceful, sweeping over you with irresistible power, or it may come in little waves. Many feel the urge as the contraction builds rather than at its onset and may wish to push only at the crest of the wave. In addition, the bearing-down urge often varies from one contraction to another.

If you don't feel the urge after the cervix is fully dilated, wait awhile. Meanwhile try relaxing, squatting for a few contractions, and the *Opening Flower* imagery.

Let your body be your guide about when and how to push.

Think of opening, not just bearing down. Janet Kingsepp of the Association of Texas Midwives tells her clients to "imagine the baby coming down while you open from the inside, being soft and loose and open." You can try this or use the *Opening Flower* imagery.

Meanwhile, tell yourself, "Let go, open, open, open."

Second stage is often more efficient if the mother grunts or just lets her breath out while she pushes. You may prefer vocalizing in other ways, even hollering. Don't hold back. Avoid holding your breath unless you feel the need.

Milestones of Second Stage

For most parents second stage is tremendously exciting. The following are some of the most memorable landmarks as the moment of birth dawns:

The father's first sight of the baby's head. "I can see the baby! I can see the baby!" exclaimed one father when he first saw what looked like a bit of matted hair at the end of a fleshy tunnel. The mother's enthusiasm about bearing down often doubles when her partner makes this dramatic announcement.

The mother's first sight of the baby's head. The father (or friend) should hold a mirror so the mother can see the baby emerging, but not insist that she view the birth if she doesn't want to. Many mothers who plan witnessing the birth through a mirror are so caught up in the overwhelming sensations of second stage that they forget all about it. This also holds true for some fathers. Though in my book *Sharing Birth: A Father's Guide to Giving Support During Labor,* I recommend that all fathers hold a mirror for their partner during birth, my wife Jan reminds me that I forgot to do this myself!

Touching the baby's head while it is still inside. "What a strange thrill it was feeling something in me that was not me!" Eva exclaimed, recalling touching her baby's head before it crowned. This can be an especially tender moment in the childbearing drama. The father can remind her, "Reach down and touch our baby."

Crowning. As already stated, many mothers experience a burning or splitting sensation as the largest diameter of the baby's head passes through the birth outlet. Some actually experience orgasm. A threshold experience, crowning can be a moment of panic. But it passes quickly.

Your caregiver will probably tell you to stop pushing and either to pant or blow so the head will ease out without your tearing. Meanwhile, your partner can tell you to "open like a flower."

Completing the Rite of Passage

When your baby is born, moist from her watery home, with patches of vernix (a cheesy white substance with the consistency of luxurious hand cream), no one has to tell you how to feel or what to do.

But here is a nice way to welcome your baby. When the cord stops pulsing, your partner can cut it while you hold your child. There is nothing to this. One simply snips the cord with a pair of scissors. It is not painful to the mother or baby.

While the cord is being cut you can, if you want, both say aloud or silently in your heart: "Welcome to our home," or an equivalent.

Effective Labor Support

"The father is worth his weight in Demerol!" declare the authors of *Maternity Nursing.*[2] There is no more effective way of relieving the fear and pain of labor than his presence and support.

As the *inner event of labor* unfolds and the *heart brain* takes over, loving support is one of the laboring woman's greatest needs. In fact, it is probably as important as all the eight steps in this book combined. Nurturing support can create the conditions for the mother to surrender to labor whether she is at home or in the hospital.

Though anyone, male or female, can give effective labor support, the father is uniquely qualified for this role because he knows his partner in ways no one else does. Accordingly, this section is addressed to fathers. But whoever plans to support a woman in labor will find it helpful.

The Father's Role

Many childbirth professionals refer to a laboring woman's partner as a "labor coach." But this is a misleading term. The father should avoid seeing himself in this light. Birth is not an athletic event. He is not a coach. He is his partner's lover and the father of their child. Essentially his role during labor is twofold: to share the birth and to provide emotional and physical support.

"My world consisted of my labor and my partner," one mother said. "Nothing else mattered." Though the father too is experiencing the life-altering event of labor, it is the mother who must cope with the physiological process. Therefore he will have greater strength and be able to share it with her during labor's vulnerable moments.

Understanding the *inner event of labor* and the fact that labor is a sexual experience is an important step in providing appropriate support. In addition, the father should keep in mind the five essentials of a positive image of birth, as his image of birth will affect his confidence in the labor process and the kind of support he gives. Accordingly, he should read thoroughly chapters two and three.

Giving Support

Following are the basic points to keep in mind. (Additional ways to relieve the fear and pain of labor are discussed in *Sharing*

Birth: A Father's Guide to Giving Support During Labor. The father should read this book in advance of labor and have it with him as a reference at the place of birth.)

Be there and share the experience. That's the most important thing. Your presence and encouragement are worth more than anything else.

Guide her through imagery, using any or all of the exercises in this chapter or others she finds helpful.

Sit close and speak in a soothing, calm voice as you guide her.

Don't be hesitant about repetition (unless the mother dislikes it). "Open, open, open, see yourself opening like a flower, petal by petal, open, open. . . ." is quite effective for some.

Some laboring women also find repetitive chanting helpful with or without the background of relaxing music. One mother simply repeated "O-o-open" somewhat like a meditator chants "om." You can chant with her if you wish.

Be aware of signs of tension. If she tenses a hand, arm, shoulder, and so forth, tell her to relax the tense area. You can touch the area and say, "Relax toward my hand."

Massage her, paying special attention to any area that is tense or uncomfortable.

Blanket her with love. Love is the foundation of effective labor support. Expressing your love physically as well as verbally is more important than anything else at this time. Hug her, caress her.

Bear in mind that labor is a sexual event. As Elisabeth Bing points out, "The relationship between labor and lovemaking is hard to remember in the hospital environment."[3] However, it is not sensual behavior that is inappropriate during labor—it is the hospital setting.

Regardless of what is shown in many childbirth films, the best place for the father is not sitting or standing by, timing contractions while the mother labors. Rather, it is on the labor bed with her or up walking with her.

If you are in a hospital, let go. Shut the door. Tell the staff you prefer to be alone with your partner, if you wish.

If at times during labor the mother doesn't want to be touched, don't feel offended. This is normal and the way many women react in the late active phase.

Ask for feedback from time to time (between, not during, contractions). "Does this feel good? Does this help?" Following her lead, you can vary what you do to make her comfortable.

Encourage her to surrender to her sea of sensations, to let go, to open, to say yes to labor. Welcome her uninhibited behavior as a positive sign.

Encourage her to express herself freely. The laboring woman may sigh, moan, and groan, making sounds much like a woman nearing sexual climax. An effective way to work with contractions and release tension, this also indicates that she is attuned to her instinctive self.

Don't insist she breathe a certain way through labor unless she finds this helpful. Her own body should always be her guide. If, however, she finds previously learned breathing patterns an effective means of coping with contractions, breathe with her, guiding her breathing as necessary.

Forget the clock. "Babies don't know about calendars and due dates," states California midwife June Whitson. "Babies don't care about averages. Turn off the clock in your head and just work from one contraction to the next." The averages listed in this chapter are only *averages.* The stages of normal labor may be much longer or shorter.

Help your partner take a warm bath or shower if she wishes. Water is soothing, relaxing, a primal element. In fact, the baby is immersed in water throughout pregnancy. Some women become so relaxed in a warm tub that they don't want to leave and give birth under water. An azure pool at the maternity hospital in Pithiviers, France, is set up just for this purpose. She can do imagery in the tub.

A shower with water running over the belly and back is also quite relaxing. The mother can imagine herself giving her tension to the water, letting it flow away.

Apply facecloths (or towels) soaked in very warm water and wrung dry to the area of discomfort: the lower belly, the lower back, the thighs, the area between the vagina and anus, and so forth.

If the mother panics there are two effective ways to calm her. If she is screaming, suggest that she lower the pitch of her voice and groan. This tends to dissolve fear. If you want, groan with her.

You can also suggest she breathe with you, and guide her breathing. Keep up eye contact and be firm if needed.

Should a cesarean be necessary, being at your partner's side is especially important. A screen placed between your partner's head and abdomen blocks your view of the surgery. If you want to observe the birth, you can simply stand up. After birth, unless the baby requires immediate pediatric attention, you can hold the baby close so both of you can see and touch her.

If the mother is frightened that what she is experiencing is abnormal, tell the caregiver. The caregiver can reassure her or cope with the problem if there is one.

Meanwhile, realize that giving birth is an awesome experience. At times it can be emotionally and physically overwhelming. It is all right to be afraid.

The father too may feel helpless and frightened at times. This is perfectly normal. After all, you are both taking part in a miracle as great as the creation of the earth.

And who can stand before the Creator and not tremble?

∽ CHAPTER TEN

Enjoying the First Hours after Birth:
THE EIGHTH STEP

The moment has finally come.

The baby has emerged from a cushioned watery home to the parents' waiting arms.

The mother explores her child with her eyes, her fingertips; she enfolds him in her arms close to her skin.

The baby explores his mother with his eyes. He roots for the nipple.

The father takes the moist tiny child in his arms. He gazes into his child's eyes.

The baby looks back into his father's eyes.

It is magic.

Few moments equal that first tremendous greeting between parents and child. After the baby is born, you may feel a burst of energy, waves of elation and joy. Or you may simply be exhausted and relieved. Initial uncertainty is also normal when first seeing your child. In any case, this time is special, and spending it together without interruptions in an emotionally positive climate is an important aspect of concluding a normal birth.

A New Family Is Born

Many children's books depict ridiculous scenes with one or more objects that don't belong there—a snowman on the beach on a hot summer day, a giant lizard in a three-piece suit walking down Wall Street with the rush-hour commuters, and so on. The child's job is to find what's out of place.

Often modern childbirth scenes contain elements as ridiculous as the Wall Street lizard. For example, a mother lies on a stainless steel table while her baby is on the other side of the room in a clear plastic bassinet being frightened half to death by busy attendants. Clearly something is out of place.

It's obvious—even to a tiny child—where the baby belongs after birth.

A Time for Love

The first hour after birth is a time for love, not clinical procedures. Unless there are rare complications requiring emergency medical care, the baby belongs in the parents' arms, perhaps more so now than at any other time.

Like labor, the immediate postpartum period is an emotionally sensitive time. Following a natural birth, the baby and mother will probably be alert, particularly receptive to one another. The ongoing process of parent-infant attachment (bonding) now unfolds.

In a natural setting uninterrupted by clinical procedures, both mothers and fathers greet their babies with specific behavior which is believed to strengthen the parent-child bond. For the new mother, this includes eye contact, a pattern of touch usually beginning with fingertip exploration of the child's head and extremities, caressing the baby with the palm, and then enfolding the baby in her arms.

For the father, the first moment of eye contact is often the most beautiful and overwhelming of the entire childbearing experience. The new father often feels elated and exhilarated as he holds and becomes engrossed with his child.

Nothing should interrupt the new family during this time. All routine medical procedures—prophylactic eyedrops to prevent gonococcal-caused blindness, the newborn exam, and so forth— should be delayed at least one hour. Then, the baby can be examined at your side.

The steps in this book—developing a positive image of birth, understanding the *inner event of labor*, choosing a good caregiver and appropriate birthing place—apply as much to the first hours after birth as to labor. They will eliminate emotional trauma for you and your child, provided the birth is normal, and affect the way you feel throughout the six-week postpartum period.

As already stated, the birthing place should be one where you not only feel medically safe, but where you are comfortable beginning a family. An environment conducive to the *inner event of labor* is most conducive to parent-infant attachment.

The mother is particularly sensitive to her environment during the first hours following birth just as she is in labor. An overly clinical, emotionally negative atmosphere or insensitive staff can interfere with bonding with her child, her ability to breastfeed, and her expression of normal feelings that follow birth.

Both parents and childbirth professionals are becoming increasingly aware of the significance of the first hours after birth. Many hospital maternity units and childbearing centers offer a positive emotional climate for those who aren't comfortable with birthing at home. The widespread use of the central nursery is waning. The practice of separating mothers and babies is falling by the wayside as more and more childbirth professionals rediscover that birth is not a medical procedure but a natural life event. However, in a few hospitals mothers and babies are routinely separated immediately or shortly after birth. The baby is whisked away to an infant warmer for medical procedures, then to a nursery.

Such a bizarre custom can have a shattering effect on mother and newborn. One cannot interfere with a natural process so powerful yet so delicate without consequences. Removing the baby from the mother is both traumatic for the child and also probably the single most significant cause of postpartum depression or *baby blues*. This is yet another reason to choose your caregiver and birthing place carefully.

Bear in mind that normal mothers have a wide range of reactions after birth, from "I was so excited I couldn't sit down!" to "All I wanted to do was sleep!" If you don't experience immediate elation, it doesn't mean anything is wrong.

The same applies if the first few hours are interrupted by unforeseen circumstances. Parent-infant attachment is an ongoing process. Though spending the first few hours together is the *normal* way to follow a natural birth, missing this time will in no way interfere with your being a good parent or loving your child.

Essentials for the First Hours After Birth

The following will contribute toward a smoother transition to parenthood and help you make the most of the time you spend with your child immediately after birth.

Take the baby immediately to breast. Nursing is an important part of normal birth for both the baby and the mother. The premilk fluid, colostrum, contains the precise nutrients your baby requires as well as immune factors to resist a host of infections.

For the mother, nursing causes the release of the hormone oxytocin. This causes the uterus to contract, facilitating the delivery of the placenta and clamping down on blood vessels at the placental site, thereby helping to prevent postpartum hemorrhage.

Nursing shortly after birth is so important that I believe every mother (birthing vaginally or surgically) should attempt it, whether or not she plans to breastfeed later.

Most babies will take the breast immediately. But don't be

concerned if your baby doesn't. This is also perfectly normal. Some babies need encouragement (putting the nipple in the baby's mouth or squirting a few drops on his tongue) or simply patience.

Hold the baby close, skin to skin, both parents. Immediate and prolonged parent-infant contact is a dramatic and wonderful follow-up to birth.

Be sure the room is dimly lit. Nothing should interfere with that wondrous eye contact that follows birth. It will take some time for the baby to get used to bright lights. If the baby is born surgically in a brightly lit delivery room, the father can cup his hands a little above the baby's eyes to encourage the baby to open them.

Involve siblings immediately or very shortly after birth. If the children don't attend the birth, meeting the newborn shortly afterward may lessen trauma and make emotional adjustment easier. Children too need to adjust to the life-altering event of having a baby.

If you give birth out of your home, consider early discharge. Typically, new mothers leave childbearing centers within twenty-four hours. There is no reason you can't do the same if you birth in a hospital, provided everything is normal. Adjusting to parenthood is easier in your own surroundings and in the presence of family and friends.

If your baby needs immediate medical care and must be taken to an intensive care unit, accompany the newborn. Should the mother be unable to move right away, the father can go to the intensive care unit and share the child's first hours with the mother later.

If you have had cesarean surgery, pay special attention to spending time with the baby and to your partner's help and support. Rooming in with the baby will facilitate breastfeeding and parent-infant attachment. The father's support will lessen trauma while the mother is in the unique role of needing to be cared for as well as taking on her own caretaking role.

(Further information about the period immediately following birth, including the father's unique role after cesarean surgery, is covered in my book *After the Baby Is Born.*)

The Baby Blues

"Over 80 percent of women giving birth in hospitals in the United States suffer from postpartum blues," states anthropologist Ashley Montagu.[1] Postpartum depression or "baby blues" is a constellation of stress, irritability, fatigue, and tears that most often appears between the third and fifth day after birth and may last from a few days to several weeks. This phenomenon is so common that many health professionals believe it is an almost inevitable consequence of giving birth.

Once the baby is born, both parents have new and irreversible roles. You have crossed the one-way bridge to parenthood. This is bound to cause stress and a certain amount of negative emotion, especially during the first weeks. But prolonged baby blues is not inevitable. If all your plans reflect the five essentials of a positive image of birth and are conducive to the *inner event of labor,* you will decrease considerably your chance of getting baby blues. This is because the baby blues is largely the result of unnatural birth customs. In fact, according to Ashley Montagu, "The principal cause of postpartum blues is separation of the baby from the mother."[2]

Postpartum depression is significantly less common after home births. Aidan Macfarlane, pediatrician and author of *The Psychology of Childbirth,* states, "In one study, the figures were that some depression occurred in 60 percent of hospital deliveries and in only 16 percent of home deliveries."[3] Presumably the reason for this tremendous difference is that at home, natural parental behavior is not interrupted and mother and baby are never separated.

Going home shortly after birth is almost always the best course of action unless there are medical problems. If you are in a clinical setting, early discharge is especially beneficial to mother, father, and baby's emotional well-being. According to Helen Varney, author of *Nurse-Midwifery*, early discharge from a hospital that has inflexible policies and routinely practices maternal-infant separation "decreases the incidence and severity of postpartum blues."

The hospital can sometimes provide an environment conducive to beginning a family and eliminating unnecessary depression. Dr. Michel Odent observes that postpartum depression is rare at the Pithiviers maternity unit (in France), where birth is approached as a wholly natural event and medical procedures don't interrupt parent-infant contact. Though childbearing centers and hospitals can provide positive emotional climates for new families, the environment can, of course, never match that of home.

Welcoming the Baby

Doing this imagery will help both parents prepare for birth as well as the time shortly following. It gives your inner mind a goal: enjoying your baby after a rewarding birth. Although this is a perfectly obvious goal of pregnancy, creating this scene in the mind's eye "programs" you to achieve the goal.

Get into a comfortable position and relax.

Imagine being with your child after birth. Create in your mind's eye the scene you really want to experience.

See yourself exploring your new baby, welcoming your child to your home.

If anything seems out of place, rearrange the image until you have created the scene that feels right.

Tell yourself: I am enjoying this time after birth in the best possible way for myself and my baby.

When you are ready, slowly count to five, stretch gently, and open your eyes.

The Inner Event of Nursing

With rare exceptions, anyone who can give birth can nurse her child. Today most childbirth professionals and pediatricians realize that mother's milk is the only perfectly designed and truly safe food for baby. The majority of parents interested in natural childbirth choose to breastfeed.

Like both labor and lovemaking, nursing is influenced by the mother's attitude, her emotions, and her environment. The mother nurses best when she is relaxed, emotionally at ease, and well supported.

The basics of successful nursing are:

- Good nutrition and adequate fluids
- A supportive partner
- Relaxation
- A positive attitude
- A supportive caregiver.

Two fundamental processes are involved in nursing: the baby's sucking and the let-down, or milk-ejection reflex (the name of this reflex was borrowed from dairy farmers who speak of cows "letting down" the milk). When the baby sucks the breast, oxytocin is released by the pituitary gland in the brain, causing cells around the alveoli (milk-producing lobes) and cells surrounding milk ducts leading from those lobes to the nipple to contract. This pushes the milk through the ducts to little reservoirs, called milk sinuses, under the nipple. The let-down may also be triggered and the breasts actually begin to leak milk even before the baby sucks—when the baby cries or when the mother just thinks of the baby.

"The let-down reflex is a simple physical response to a physical stimulus," Karen Pryor explains in *Nursing Your Baby*. "Why then is failure of the let-down reflex the basic cause of almost every breastfeeding failure? Because this reflex is greatly affected by the mother's emotions."[4]

If the mother is anxious, upset, or in the presence of someone critical of nursing, the milk may not let down freely.[5] For example, the first six weeks after birth, Sarah found it difficult to nurse her baby boy. Her husband was away much of the time on business and she stayed with his parents, who were skeptical of breastfeeding. Almost every time she nursed, they expressed disapproval. "All our children were bottle fed," they said, or "The baby looks thin. Are you sure he's well nourished?"

Sarah's milk wouldn't "let down" and she too began to worry that her baby wasn't getting enough. She had all but turned to bottle feeding when her husband decided to spend more time with her and the baby. The new parents also confronted the critical grandparents and asked them to respect their way of feeding the child. Almost immediately, the nursing problem vanished and the milk let down freely.

We've discussed how profoundly one's image of birth affects the labor process and the overall experience of childbearing. Developing a positive image is perhaps the most important step the expectant parents can take toward a safe, rewarding birth. The same holds for nursing. The way both mother and father feel about nursing will greatly influence whether or not nursing is successful.

In my book *After the Baby is Born* I urge both parents to be involved in the nursing decision. Nursing is not likely to be entirely satisfying if either partner has strong negative feelings about it. A supportive partner is a crucial element in successful nursing. The father's attitude can spell the difference between breastfeeding success or failure.

Some parents make a decision against nursing as a result either of negative feelings or myths about the subject. Exploring and letting go of these during pregnancy or, if necessary, after the baby is born can make a tremendous difference.

Is the baby really getting enough food? This is an objection often voiced by relatives several years ago and less commonly today. Now more and more people realize that the supply adjusts to the demand. Nursing is, in fact, the only way to ensure that the baby is getting all the nutrients he really needs.

Will nursing ruin our sexual relationship? Nursing mothers do have varying reactions to lovemaking—from increased to decreased desire. But in either case, if the couple is close they can always find ways to fulfill one another's needs. Nursing never contraindicates lovemaking.

However, some fathers do have to learn to see the breasts performing a utilitarian as well as a sexual function. They may have to learn to share the breast with the baby.

Many fathers feel jealous when the mother nurses. After all, the baby is now the center of attention, receiving so much love and affection. Feelings of jealousy are often worsened if the mother, perhaps as a result of the normal exhaustion that follows birth, pays less attention to her partner.

However, with consideration on the part of both parents, jealousy can usually be easily overcome. Perhaps the most important thing is making time to be alone with one another. I believe it is essential to make arrangements to spend time without the baby during the first few weeks and months of parenthood— even if it's just for an occasional hour or evening.

Some parents are concerned that breastfeeding will restrict their freedom. Nursing does carry certain built-in obligations. For example, either the baby must be breastfed or, if the mother is not with the baby, she must periodically express her milk.

But the inconveniences of nursing are slight compared to those of bottle feeding: buying, washing, and sterilizing bottles, to say nothing of warming the 2 A.M. feeding. Furthermore, breastfeeding has advantages that far outweigh its disadvantages, in addition to numerous health benefits for the baby. The food is always at the perfect temperature; it is much less expensive; diapers are less odorous; and mother can feed the baby anytime, anywhere, with no preparation whatever.

In addition, breastfeeding need not be an all or nothing affair. Though I personally recommend 100 percent breastfeeding, many couples supplement nursing quite satisfactorily—for instance, if the mother works throughout the day. In any case, breast milk supplemented with formula is far better than no breast milk at all.

Many breastfeeding problems and negative feelings can probably be blamed on societal attitudes. Cultural conditioning can influence breastfeeding just as it affects childbearing. For example, in cultures where nursing is almost 100 percent successful, the prevailing social attitude is entirely supportive of nursing. Among the Aymara of Bolivia, "No modesty is attached to nursing even in public places," Niles Newton observes. "Nursing has precedence over any other activity in which the mother may be engaged, such as selling her vegetables in the market, for instance, although she may be extremely anxious to make the sale."[6] And in Jordan, "Both in everyday life and at the festivals one can observe how, as soon as the child cries or shows the least sign of restlessness, it is at once laid to the mother's breast. Very often a woman who is nursing a child has an opening in her dress over each breast and thus she can feed it at once. And she does it unhesitatingly in any place at any time and very often."[7]

Our own society presents a poor comparison. Though increasing numbers of mothers nurse their babies, society as a whole is not yet entirely supportive of it. Many mothers and fathers go through their entire prechildbearing lives never having seen a mother breastfeeding. Nursing is still a relative rarity in parks and other public places, while feeding a child a bottle is a common sight! This is yet another Wall Street lizard of childbearing.

Fortunately, however, a saner, healthier, happier view is emerging. It is hoped that this book will further help a more positive image of childbearing and breastfeeding to evolve.

Meanwhile, the steps in *Mind Over Labor* will help you to surround your experience of childbearing and nursing with love.

Using Relaxation and Imagery

Relaxation is the key to successful nursing. In this imagery, you are focusing your mind on images that suggest flowing to influence the breast milk to flow.

Get into a comfortable position and relax.

Imagine yourself in your *special place.*

Now tell yourself: I am able to supply all my baby's nutritional needs to grow and be perfectly healthy.

At this point you can use any number of images that appeal to you—a waterfall, a geyser, a flowing stream, a meadow clothed in wildflowers with a brook running through it—anything that suggests flowing.

When you are ready, slowly count to five, stretch gently, and open your eyes.

Any of the relaxation exercises in chapter four will also help nursing.

Appendix:

Using Mental Imagery for Special Situations

Pregnancy and childbirth do not always progress smoothly. Problems occasionally arise even under the best circumstances.

Good nutrition, regular exercise, and careful observation of all the eight steps in this book will minimize your chance of complications. However, should complications nevertheless arise in pregnancy, labor or after birth, you can use relaxation and mental imagery for healing. According to Dr. Mike Samuels and Nancy Samuels in *The Well Baby Book*, "Visualizing healing images results in general body changes, including muscle relaxation, changed blood flow, decreased oxygen consumption and output of metabolic waste products, lowered respiration and heart rate, easier breathing and decreased awareness of pain." The authors point out that specific imagery can produce even more radical changes, such as increased blood flow to a particular area to speed the healing of an infection.[1]

The simplest and probably most universal healing image involves going into a deep state of relaxation and imagining yourself surrounded with a white or golden light. If you wish, you can imagine brilliant sunlight filling your entire being, or imagine that the light is creative or divine energy.

Following are additional images and other remedies for specific problems:

Turning a Breech

In the *breech* position the buttocks or feet rather than the head are born first. If your baby is breech, your caregiver will usually discover this and let you know by the eighth month.

"During pregnancy I believed it wasn't good for a baby to be upside down," remarked one mother after a breech birth. "I often wonder if that influenced his position." It's hard to say whether or not this mother's thoughts influenced her baby's position in the uterus.

Many physicians do cesareans for all breech babies. Others are familiar with handling a breech birth naturally or will attempt turning the baby manually with hands on the abdomen.

You can try to influence the baby's position by using a combination of position and mental imagery. Dr. Juliet M. DeSouza has found the mother's physical position alone 89 percent successful for turning a breech baby. [2]

Lie flat on your back with knees bent, feet flat on the floor, with pillows or cushions under the buttocks so the pelvis is nine to twelve inches off the floor.

Imagine the baby floating in fluid, head down and comfortably resting on a little pillow of crystal-clear water.

Or (as suggested by Suzanna May Hilbers), imagine children tumbling and turning somersaults, or clothes turning over in the dryer, to facilitate the baby's turning.

Vaginal Birth after a Previous Cesarean

Today we realize that the old dictum "Once a cesarean, always a cesarean" is not valid. If you have had a cesarean section in the past and are now planning a vaginal birth, you are just as likely to birth naturally as anyone else, provided there are no medical complications with *this* pregnancy. However, you should take certain precautions to increase your chance of birthing normally:

- Choose a caregiver who recognizes that your condition is *normal.*
- Choose a birthing place with all the essential qualities listed in chapter seven.
- Avoid *all* unnecessary medical intervention.
- Pay special attention to labor support. Your partner's help is especially important in keeping you feeling positive— particularly if you are laboring in a hospital.
- Use imagery that makes you feel confident and strong and inspires trust in the body and the normal process of labor.
- Use affirmations with relaxation and imagery to remind yourself that you are able to birth naturally.

If a Cesarean Is Necessary

In rare circumstances, cesarean surgery is unavoidable. Mixed emotions often follow the birth. While at first the new parents may experience the elation that so often crowns the reproductive miracle, disappointment, tears, and anger may follow.

After a cesarean, both partners have a much harder beginning to parenthood than those who have birthed normally. The mother must recover from major abdominal surgery as well as from having given birth. She must adopt a caretaking role at the same time that she is in the position of needing care. The father will have the additional burden of taking care of his partner and baby.

He can help tremendously by taking extra paternity leave to spend time in the hospital with the mother and baby and later help out at home.

Meanwhile, rooming in with the baby and breastfeeding as soon as possible after birth are especially important, even though it may be difficult for the mother. These vital measures will facilitate parent-infant attachment, help both mother and baby minimize the trauma of surgery, and make the smoothest possible transition to parenthood under the circumstances. For more about cesarean recovery and making the most of the first few weeks after birth, see my book *After the Baby Is Born*.

Both parents should discuss their feelings. Allow yourselves to grieve if you feel sad about not having had a vaginal birth. Grieving is part of the healing process.

Unfortunately, some health professionals are unaware of the intense feelings many cesarean parents experience. See the references at the end of this book. From time to time the parents may have to remind themselves that though a cesarean section is major surgery, it is also the birth of a child.

This imagery may help the healing process:

Imagine the stitched site in your mind's eye. Picture the area healing perfectly. See yourself moving about without discomfort. Tell yourself that healing is taking place faster than you expected.

Induced Labor

Babies are rarely born on schedule. The due date is only an estimate and accurate about 5 percent of the time. Expect the baby a week or two before or after.

If, however, labor is more than a couple of weeks overdue or there is an illness such as preeclampsia (a pregnancy illness in which there is increased blood pressure and excessive fluid retention) or diabetes, your caregiver may suggest induction. "There are medical indications for inducing labor which are undoubtably life-saving," writes the pediatrician Aidan Macfarlane in *The Psychology of Childbirth*, "and in these cases it is obvious that any detrimental emotional or behavioral effects will be of secondary importance."[3]

The two medical methods of inducing labor are artificial rupture of the membranes (amniotomy) and the administration of intravenous Pitocin solution, a form of the hormone oxytocin which helps to initiate and regulate contractions.

However, both carry risks. Rupturing the membranes, according to Dr. Roberto Caldeyro-Barcia, the former president of the International Federation of Gynecologists and Obstetricians and director of the Latin American Center for Perinatology and Human Development for the World Health Organization, may risk increasing pressure on the baby's head and umbilical cord, causing fetal distress and resulting in a cesarean. Furthermore, an amniotomy sets the labor clock in motion, as many hospitals require a woman to give birth within twenty-four hours after membranes have ruptured (owing to increased risk of infection).

Pitocin generally causes more painful contractions, with increased need for pain medication. In addition, the baby is at higher risk of becoming jaundiced.

Unless there is an emergency, natural means should be tried before resorting to medical induction. (Check with your caregiver before trying them.) These include:

- Hiking, jogging. Walking is a well-known way to speed up a flagged labor and may also initiate contractions.
- Eating spicy, gas-producing foods (such as chili or pizza) and drinking carbonated beverages. The hyperactive intestines may trigger contractions. (The precise way this works is unknown.)
- Lovemaking (do not have intercourse if the bag of waters has broken) and oral or manual nipple stimulation. Orgasm can trigger uterine contractions *if* the cervix is ripe (soft and partially effaced) and the mother is ready for labor. Nipple stimulation causes the release of oxytocin, which may cause contractions. You can stimulate your own nipples by massaging with hot moist washcloths.
- Discuss any concerns you have about birth, becoming a

mother, and so on, with your partner. Emotional conflicts are often responsible for an overdue labor.

- Use mental imagery. Try *Talking with Your Baby* (pages 87–89) and ask your child what is holding her back; *The Special Place,* imagining that you have already given birth and are with your child, happy; and *The Opening Flower.*

Prolonged Labor

The length of labor varies widely. Usually it is best to forget the clock. However, should labor seem overly long, there are several things to try.

For First Stage
For early labor: (cervix dilated less than 3 to 5 cm.)

It is usually unnecessary to do anything about a prolonged early phase. Contractions may simply come and fade as time passes. Just continue with your daily life and get plenty of rest.

However, if contractions are persistent and not dilating the cervix and you have difficulty sleeping, you can try: relaxing, taking a bath or shower, or a change of environment (if in the hospital, consider going home or outdoors). You might also distract yourself by visiting friends, taking a walk, watching TV, and so forth.

For active labor: (cervix dilated more than 4 to 5 cm.)

If contractions fade once labor has become active, there are several things to try:

- Rest or sleep until labor resumes activity.
- Relax.
- Bathe or shower.
- Massage.
- Drink sweet liquids to restore your energy and body fluids (tea with honey, fruit juice, and so on).

- Walk.
- Change position.
- Make love (no intercourse if membranes have ruptured) and/or nipple stimulation.
- Change your environment. If a particular person is making you uncomfortable, ask that person to leave you alone for a while. If the environment itself is making you uncomfortable, try turning down the lights, playing soft music, and doing *The Special Place* (pages 70–71).
- Talk about concerns you have about birth and parenthood.
- Mental imagery: *The Special Place, The Opening Flower, Imagining the Birth,* and any others you find relaxing.

Staff persons, family and/or friends in the birthing room can sometimes interfere with the mother's labor. This is especially true if those present are impatient for labor to move along. The mother may feel that she must perform in a certain way, which can inhibit her from letting go and laboring normally. (Psychotherapist and childbirth counselor Gayle Peterson calls this "performance anxiety.")

The simple remedy is to ask everyone (including hospital staff) to leave for a while. This frequently clears the field emotionally and labor gets going again. You can always ask people to come back once labor picks up or when the head is ready to be born.

Sometimes the father's presence inhibits the labor process, especially if he is unsupportive, very nervous, or if there is tension between the partners. This is a delicate issue, as one can't very well ask the father to leave. However, a sensitive caregiver or nurse can help him calm down. Or he can leave for a short while until labor picks up.

For second stage:

Once the cervix is fully dilated, most babies are born within one-half to four hours. However, the relative difficulty, length, and discomfort of second stage vary depending on a number of factors, including the size and position of your baby.

To help a long second-stage progress:

- Change positions. Try standing or squatting to enlist the aid of gravity.
- Use *The Opening Flower* or *Imagining the Birth.*

A Posterior Baby

In this position, the back of the baby's skull presses against the mother's spine and may cause back pain (back labor) and a prolonged second stage.

To alleviate:

- Try positions that keep the baby's head off the spine: squatting, hands and knees, standing or kneeling, and leaning forward against partner or bed.
- During contractions your partner can apply back counter-pressure with the heel of his hand against your spine, adjusting pressure as desired.
- Imagine the contractions are ocean waves gently rocking the baby, then rolling him over.

Newborns in Intensive Care

Newborns may need medical attention for a variety of reasons. Premature babies, for instance, need special care and the baby is usually placed in a special nursery or intensive care unit (ICU).

If your baby has to be in the ICU, be sure to spend time with her—especially the first few hours after birth. Being together shortly after birth is particularly important if there are problems.

You may find it reassuring to talk with other parents in similar situations. Many hospitals hold informal meetings for such parents. "It is worth noting," writes pediatrician Aidan Macfarlane in *The Psychology of Childbirth*, "that parents of premature babies, when asked what kind of help they needed and wanted, were given a choice of doctors, social workers, psychologists, family and friends. But their choice was other parents who had themselves been separated from their children."[4]

Using mental imagery and beaming healing energy to your child may facilitate healing. Parents and children are closely linked in ways science doesn't understand. According to Mike and Nancy Samuels, "This powerful psychic connection between parents and baby probably allows for greater ease in transmission of healing images and their energy."[5]

You can do this imagery in the presence of the baby or at a distance.

Imagine the baby well, radiating health and strength.
Imagine light and love completely surrounding the baby.
You can also picture illness as a dark color flowing away.

Notes

Chapter 1. Mind Over Labor

1. Carl O. Simonton, Stephanie Matthews Simonton, and James L. Creighton, *Getting Well Again* (New York: Bantam, 1981), 26–27.

2. Herbert Benson, *The Relaxation Response* (New York: Avon, 1975), 162.

3. David Stewart and Lee Stewart, eds., *21st Century Obstetrics Now!* vol. 1 (Marble Hill, MO: NAPSAC, Inc., 1977), 63.

4. Ibid.

5. Ibid.

6. Ibid.

7. Ibid.

8. Ibid., p. 62.

9. Noble, Elizabeth, *Childbirth With Insight* (Boston: Houghton Mifflin Co., 1983), 79.

10. Elkins, Valmai Howe, *The Birth Report* (Toronto: Lester and Orpen Dennys, 1983), 45.

11. Stewart and Stewart, *21st Century Obstetrics Now!* vol. 1; A. J. Crandon, "Maternal anxiety and obstetric complications," *Journal of Psychosomatic Research* 23:109–111; R. L. McDonald, "The role of emotional factors in obstetrical complications: a review," *Psychosomatic Medicine* 30:222–243; R. L. McDonald and A. C. Christakos, "Relationship of emotional factors during pregnancy to obstetrical complications," *American Journal of Obstetrics and Gynecology* 86:341–8; and N. Uddenberg, et al., "Reproductive Conflicts: Mental Symptoms during Pregnancy and Time in Labor," *Journal of Psychosomatic Research* 20 (1976):575–81.

12. Niles Newton, "Clinical Psychoneuroendocrinology in Reproduction, Proceedings of the Second Symposium," vol. 22, L. Carenza, P. Pancheri, and L. Zichella, eds. (London: Academic Press, 1978), 415.

13. David Stewart, *The Five Standards for Safe Childbearing* (Marble Hill, MO: NAPSAC,1981), 176.

14. Newton, "Psychoneuroendocrinology."

15. Karen Pryor, *Nursing Your Baby* (New York: Pocket Books, 1975).

16. J. K. Burns, "Proceedings: relationship between blood levels of cortisol and duration of human labour," *Journal of Physiology* 254:12; R. P. Lederman, E. Lederman, B. A. Work, and D. C. McCann, "The relationship of maternal anxiety, plasma catecholamines and plasma cortisol to progress in labor," *American Journal of Obstetrics and Gynecology* 132:495–500.

17. Simonton, Simonton, and Creighton, *Getting Well Again*, 26–27.

18. David Meier, "Imagine That," *Training and Development Journal* (May 1984):26.

Chapter 2. Understanding the Inner Event of Labor: The First Step

1. Grantly Dick-Read, *Childbirth Without Fear* (New York: Harper & Row, 1978), 10.

2. Gayle Peterson, *Birthing Normally* (Berkeley: Mindbody Press, 1984), 180.

3. Michel Odent, *Birth Reborn* (New York: Pantheon, 1984), 54.

4. Ibid., 47.

5. Sheila Kitzinger and John A. David, *The Place of Birth* (New York: Oxford University Press, 1978), 201.

6. Leni Schwartz, *The World of the Unborn* (New York: Marek, 1980).

7. Niles Newton, *Maternal Emotions* (New York: Paul B. Hoeber, 1982).

8. Ibid.

9. Peterson, *Birthing Normally*, 133.

10. Margaret Duncan Jensen, Ralph C. Benson, and Irene M. Bobak, *Maternity Care: The Nurse and the Family* 2d ed. (New York: C. V. Mosby Co., 1981).

11. Elisabeth Bing and Libby Colman, *Making Love During Pregnancy* (New York: Bantam, 1977), 124.

12. Emmett E. Miller, M.D., *Great Expectations* (Stanford, CA: Source, 1983).

Chapter 3. Developing a Positive Image of Birth: The Second Step

1. Nancy Wainer Cohen and Lois J. Estner, *Silent Knife* (South Hadley, MA: Bergin & Garvey, 1983).
2. Peterson, *Birthing Normally*, 4.
3. Elisabeth Bing and Libby Colman, *Making Love During Pregnancy*, 130.
4. Claudia Panuthos, *Transformation Through Birth* (South Hadley, MA: Bergin & Garvey, 1984), 27.
5. Rahima Baldwin, *Special Delivery* (Millbrae, CA: Les Femmes, 1979), 136.
6. Odent, *Birth Reborn*.
7. Cohen and Estner, *Silent Knife*, 264.
8. Diana Korte and Roberta Scaer, *A Good Birth, A Safe Birth* (New York: Bantam, 1984).
9. Cohen and Estner, *Silent Knife*, 73.
10. Ibid.
11. Elsye Birkinshaw, *Think Slim—Be Slim* (Santa Barbara, CA: Woodbridge Press, 1976).
12. Elizabeth Noble, *Childbirth with Insight* (Boston: Houghton Mifflin, 1983), 15.

Chapter 4. Relaxing Mind and Body: The Third Step

1. Dick-Read, *Childbirth Without Fear*, 34.
2. Ibid.
3. Ibid., 6.
4. Ibid., 31.
5. Edmund Jacobson, *Progressive Relaxation* (Chicago: University of Chicago Press, 1939).
6. W. Luthe, *Autogenic Therapy* (New York: Grune & Stratton, 1969).
7. Herbert Benson, M.D., *The Relaxation Response* (New York: Avon, 1975), 162.

Chapter 5. How to Use Mental Imagery

1. Simonton, Simonton, and Creighton, *Getting Well Again*.
2. Shakti Gawain, *Creative Visualization* (Mill Valley, CA: Whatever, 1978), 38–39.
3. Mike Samuels and Nancy Samuels, *Seeing with the Mind's Eye* (New York: Random House, 1975), 148.

Chapter 6. Using Mental Imagery during Pregnancy: The Fourth Step

1. Panuthos, *Transformation through Birth*.
2. Carl Jones, *Sharing Birth: A Father's Guide to Giving Support During Labor* (New York: William Morrow & Co., 1985).
3. Schwartz, *The World of the Unborn*.
4. Mike Samuels and Nancy Samuels, *The Well Baby Book* (New York: Summit Books, 1979), 64.

Chapter 7. Creating the Optimal Birthing Environment: The Fifth Step

1. Stewart and Stewart, *21st Century Obstetrics Now!* vol. 1, 62.
2. David Stewart, *The Five Standards for Safe Childbearing* (Marble Hill, MO: NAPSAC International, Inc., 1981).
3. Cited in Elkins, *The Birth Report*, 157.
4. Kitzinger and Davis, *The Place of Birth*.
5. Aidan Macfarlane, *The Psychology of Childbirth* (Cambridge: Harvard University Press, 1977), 29.
6. Helen Wessel, *Under the Apple Tree* (Fresno, CA: Bookmates, 1981).
7. Sheila Kitzinger, *The Birth Center Newsletter* (Summer 1978) issued 188 Old Street, London.
8. Stewart and Stewart, *21st Century Obstetrics Now!* vol. 1, p. 62.
9. *Wall Street Journal* (November 29, 1983).
10. Cited in Stewart and Stewart, *21st Century Obstetrics Now!* vol. 2, p. 599.
11. David Stewart, *Safe Childbearing*, 414.

Chapter 8. Invitation to a Birth: The Sixth Step

1. National Institutes of Child Health and Human Development, "Draft Report of the Task Force on Cesarean Childbirth" (Bethesda, MD: NIH, September 1980).
2. Cohen and Estner, *Silent Knife*, 9.
3. Murray Enkin, *The Cybele Report* 5 (Spring 1984):3.
4. Dick-Read, *Childbirth Without Fear*.

Chapter 9. Using Mental Imagery in Labor: The Seventh Step

1. Samuels and Samuels, *The Well Baby Book*, 56.
2. Sharon J. Reeder, Luigi Mastroianni, Jr., and Leonide L. Martin,

Maternity Nursing 14th Ed. (Philadelphia: J. B. Lippincott Co., 1980).

3. Bing and Colman, *Making Love During Pregnancy,* 124.

Chapter 10. Enjoying the First Hours after Birth: The Eighth Step

1. Stewart and Stewart, *21st Century Obstetrics Now!* vol. 2, p. 597.
2. Ibid.
3. Macfarlane, *Psychology of Childbirth,* 30.
4. Karen Pryor, *Nursing Your Baby* (New York: Pocket Books, 1975).
5. Niles Newton, "Key Psychological Issues in Human Lactation," Symposium on Human Lactation (Rockville, MD: U.S. Department of Health, Education and Welfare, Publication No. (HSA) 79-5107):29.
6. Ibid., 28.
7. Ibid., 29.

Appendix: Using Mental Imagery for Special Situations

1. Samuels and Samuels, *The Well Baby Book,* 342.
2. Baldwin, *Special Delivery.*
3. Macfarlane, *The Psychology of Childbirth.*
4. Macfarlane, *The Psychology of Childbirth.*
5. Samuels and Samuels, *The Well Baby Book,* 343.

Selected Reading List

General

Dick-Read, Grantly. *Childbirth Without Fear.* New York: Harper & Row, 1978.

Elkins, Valmai Howe. *The Birth Report.* Toronto: Lester and Orpen Dennys, 1983.

————*The Rights of the Pregnant Parent.* New York: Schocken, 1976.

Simkin, Penny, Janet Whalley, and Ann Keppler. *Pregnancy, Childbirth and the Newborn.* Deephaven, MN: Meadowbrook, 1984.

Stewart, David. *The Five Standards of Safe Childbearing.* Marble Hill, MO: NAPSAC, 1981.

Stewart, David, and Lee Stewart, eds. *21st Century Obstetrics Now!* 2 vols. Marble Hill, MO: NAPSAC, 1977. (Available through NAPSAC, Inc., P.O. Box 429, Marble Hill, MO 63764.)

Pregnancy and Childbirth

Bean, Constance A. *Methods of Childbirth.* New York: Doubleday, 1982.

Bing, Elisabeth, and Libby Coleman. *Making Love During Pregnancy.* New York: Bantam, 1977.

Kitzinger, Sheila. *The Complete Book of Pregnancy, Childbirth, and the Newborn.* New York: Alfred A. Knopf, 1983.

Simkin, Penny, Janet Whalley, and Ann Keppler. *Pregnancy, Childbirth and the Newborn,* Deephaven, MN: Meadowbrook, 1984.

Planning Your Birth

Korte, Diana, and Roberta Scaer. *A Good Birth, A Safe Birth.* New York: Bantam, 1984.

The NAPSAC Directory of Alternative Birth Services and Consumer Guide.

(Order from NAPSAC, P.O. Box 646, Marble Hill, MO 63764, $9.95.)

Simkin, Penny. *Planning Your Baby's Birth* (pamphlet). (Available through Pennypress, 1100 23rd Avenue East, Seattle, WA 98112.)

Stewart, David and Lee. *Childbirth Activities Handbook: How to Get the Childbirth Option You Want in Less Than Nine Months.* (Order from NAPSAC, P.O. Box 646, Marble Hill, MO 63764, $5.95.)

Labor Support

Jones, Carl. *Sharing Birth: A Father's Guide to Giving Support During Labor.* New York: William Morrow & Co., 1985.

Jones, Carl, Henci Goer, and Penny Simkin. *The Labor Support Guide—For Fathers, Family and Friends* (pamphlet). (Available from Pennypress, 1100 23rd Avenue East, Seattle, WA 98112.)

Cesarean Birth

Cohen, Nancy Wainer, and Lois J. Estner. *Silent Knife.* South Hadley, MA: Bergin & Garvey, 1983.

Donovan, Bonnie. *The Cesarean Birth Experience.* Boston: Beacon Press, 1978.

Norwood, Christopher. *How to Avoid a Cesarean Section.* New York: Simon & Schuster, 1984.

Young, Diony, and Charles Mahan. *Unnecessary Cesareans: Ways to Avoid Them* (pamphlet). (Available from International Childbirth Education Association, P.O. Box 20048, Minneapolis, MN 55420.)

Holistic Approach to Birth

Panuthos, Claudia. *Transformation through Birth.* South Hadley, MA: Bergin & Garvey, 1984.

Peterson, Gayle. *Birthing Normally.* Berkeley: Mindbody Press, 1984.

Home Birth

Baldwin, Rahima. *Special Delivery.* Millbrae, CA: Les Femmes, 1979.

Kitzinger, Sheila, and John A. Davis, eds. *The Place of Birth.* New York: Oxford University Press, 1978.

Sagov, Stanley E., Richard I. Feinbloom, Peggy Spindel, and Archie Brodsky. *Home Birth: A Practitioner's Guide to Birth Outside the Hospital.* Rockville, MD: Aspen Systems Corporation, 1984.

Stewart, David. *The Five Standards of Safe Childbearing.* Marble Hill, MO: NAPSAC, 1981.

The Postpartum Period

Deliquadri, Lyn, and Kati Breckenridge. *The New Mother Care.* Los Angeles: Tarcher, 1978.

Harrison, Helen, and Ann Kositsky. *The Premature Baby Book: A Parent's Guide to Coping and Caring in the First Years.* New York: St. Martin's, 1984.

Jones, Carl. *After the Baby Is Born.* New York: Dodd, Mead, 1986.

Klaus, Marshall, and John H. Kendall. *Bonding: The Beginnings of Parent-Infant Attachments.* New York: New American Library, 1983.

Samuels, Mike, and Nancy Samuels. *The Well Baby Book.* New York: Summit Books, 1979.

Breastfeeding

La Leche League. *The Womanly Art of Breastfeeding.* New York: New American Library, 1983.

Pryor, Karen. *Nursing Your Baby.* New York: Pocket Books, 1976.

For Fathers

Bitman, Sam, and Sue R. Zalk. *Expectant Fathers.* New York: Ballantine, 1981.

Greenberg, Martin. *The Birth of a Father.* New York: Continuum, 1985.

Stewart, David. *Fathering and Career: A Healthy Balance* (booklet). (Available from Pennypress, 1100 23rd Avenue East, Seattle, WA 98112.)

Midwifery

Davis, Elizabeth. *A Guide to Midwifery—Heart and Hands.* New York: Bantam, 1983.

Gaskin, Ina May. *Spiritual Midwifery.* Summertown, TN: The Book Publishing Co., 1977.

Children at Birth

Malecki, M. *Mom and Dad and I Are Having a Baby.* Seattle: Pennypress, 1979.

Anderson, Sandra Van Dam, and Penny Simkin. *Birth—Through Children's Eyes.* Seattle: Pennypress, 1981.

Periodical Publications

American Baby

The first six issues of this monthly magazine are sent free to expectant or new parents. Write to request a free six-month subscription to:

American Baby Co., 575 Lexington Avenue, New York, NY 10022.

Mothering

This quarterly publication is available for $12.00 a year. Write to: Mothering, P.O. Box 8410, Santa Fe, NM 87504.

Tapes

Great Expectations—The Joy of Pregnancy and Birthing, by Emmett Miller, M.D. One side is a guide through pregnancy from conception to delivery; the other is designed to increase confidence and promote greater relaxation and enjoyment during birth. (Available for $10.95 from Source, P.O. Box W, Stanford, CA 94305, or call 415-328-7171, or 1-800-52 TAPES in states outside of California.)

The Child Within, by Leni Schwartz, Ph.D. Six meditations for pregnant couples, to enhance the experience of pregnancy and develop a relationship with the child while it is still in the womb. (Available for $9.98 from Leni Schwartz, 325 Sanchez, Santa Fe, NM 87501.)

Relaxation and Visualization in Preparation for Childbirth, by June Whitson and Roxanne Cummings. Relaxation and imagery exercises accompanied by music. (Available for $10.95 from June Whitson, Box 95, La Honda, CA 94020.)

Welcoming Your Creation Within, by Rose Heman, R.N.C.P. The first side contains suggestions for communicating with and expressing your love for your baby before it is born. The second is a birth visualization directed at overcoming fears and negative beliefs while creating a positive, relaxed attitude for a fulfilling and loving birth experience. (Available for $12.95 from Rose Heman, R.N.C.P., P.O. Box 8168, W. Bloomfield, MI 48304.)

Index